FAST FACTS

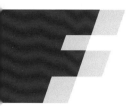

Ur(
19(

Indispensable

Guides to

Clinical

Practice

Edited by

Julian Shah

Senior Lecturer in Urology and
Consultant Urologist, Institute of Urology and
Nephrology, UCL, London, UK

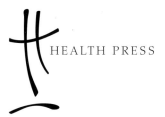

HEALTH PRESS

Oxford

Fast Facts – Urology Highlights 1997
First published 1998

© 1998 Health Press Limited
Elizabeth House, Queen Street, Abingdon,
Oxford, UK OX14 3JR
Tel: +44 (0)1235 523233
Fax: +44 (0)1235 523238

Fast Facts is a trademark of Health Press Limited

A CIP catalogue record for this title is available
from the British Library.

ISBN 1-899541-96-9

Library of Congress
Cataloging-in-Publication Data

Shah, PJR. (Julian)
Fast Facts – Urology Highlights 1997/
Julian Shah

Designed and typeset by Hinton Chaundy
Design Partnership, Thame, UK

Printed by Sterling Press, Wellingborough, UK

Contributors

Benign prostatic hyperplasia
Dr Ken Anson and Mr Roger Kirby, London

Prostate cancer
Professor Claude C Schulman and
Dr Alexander R Zlotta, Brussels

Bladder cancer
Dr Michael F Sarosdy, San Antonio

Andrology
Dr John P Mulhall and Dr Irwin Goldstein,
Boston

Urodynamics
Dr David C Chaikin and Dr Jerry G Blaivas,
New York

Incontinence
Mr Julian Shah, London

Paediatric urology
Dr Larry S Baskin, San Francisco

Neurourology
Professor Philip EV Van Kerrebroeck, Maastricht

Reconstructive urology
Mrs Suzie N Venn and Mr Anthony R Mundy,
London

Stone disease & minimally invasive surgery
Dr Francis X Keeley and Mr David A Tolley,
Edinburgh

Urinary tract infection
Dr Grannum R Sant, Boston

Introduction

Our first venture into providing up-to-date information in the field of urology for busy urologists – *Highlights 1996* – proved to be a great success. The succinct presentation of the most recent research presented at national and international meetings and published in journals in the calendar year by recognized experts in their field provides probably the most effective way to keep abreast of our ever-changing subject. What is in fashion today may not be so next year or may have been influenced by carefully controlled research; following the same format as last year, the What's In and What's Out tables complement each chapter.

Highlights 1997 continues this book series, which is intended to crystallize the advances in the year just ending. No urologist, whether those just embarking on a career or the well-experienced in the subject, should be without a copy. I hope you enjoy reading this book and will continue to collect the series.

Julian Shah
Editor

Benign prostatic hyperplasia

K Anson and R Kirby

St George's Hospital, London, UK

The past 12 months have been a period of consolidation rather than innovation in the field of benign prostatic hyperplasia (BPH).

- Our understanding of the natural history of lower urinary tract symptoms (LUTS) secondary to BPH has increased with particular interest focusing on acute urinary retention.
- The use of finasteride for prophylaxis has been proposed and the improved tolerability of the longer-acting α_1-adrenoceptor antagonists has been established.
- No major advances in the surgical management of BPH have been made, but more has been learnt about the effects of thermally-induced prostatic damage.

Natural history of LUTS and BPH

The Olmsted County community-based observational study has provided valuable information on the incidence of acute urinary retention (AUR) in men aged 40–79 years, who were followed for a mean of 50 months.[1] The overall risk of AUR was 6.8/1000 person years; risk increased with advancing age, higher American Urological Association symptom index, maximum urinary flow rate less than 12 ml/second and prostate volume of greater than 30 ml. Interestingly, 47% of episodes of AUR were associated with surgical procedures and only 13% of the men who suffered AUR (8 out of a total of 2115) underwent transurethral resection of the prostate (TURP) within 6 months.

Medical management of benign prostatic obstruction

Andersen and colleagues addressed the question of whether the 5α-reductase inhibitor, finasteride, could reduce the incidence of AUR and "BPH-related surgical interventions" in patients with significant LUTS.[2] Their pooled data analysis of a number of randomized trials, involving a total of 4222 men, showed that finasteride reduced the incidence of AUR from 2.7% to 1.1%

7

and the need for surgery from 6.5% to 4.2%. Despite the limitations of this study, it appears that finasteride, while having a modest objective symptomatic benefit in most patients, may have a future role in the prophylactic treatment of patients at risk of AUR, such as those identified in the Olmsted County data.

The α_1-adrenoceptor antagonists with a gradual onset and long duration of action have been shown to be better tolerated by patients than the shorter-acting agents.[3] Tamsulosin, the so-called 'prostate-selective' α_{1A}-blocker, has been shown to be well tolerated and effective at a single daily dose of 0.4 mg,[4] and to have a lower side-effect profile than the non-selective α_1-antagonist, terazosin.[5] While the efficacy of each drug was comparable, the improved tolerability of tamsulosin may be explained by the fact that it has an 8–35-fold higher affinity for the α_{1A}-subtype receptor, which is found in much higher concentrations in the prostate than in the extraprostatic vasculature.

Nevertheless, the non-subtype-selective adrenoceptor blockers, such as terazosin and doxazosin, still have a role to play as they lower blood pressure in hypertensive patients and about one-third of men with BPH also have concomitant hypertension. Data are also emerging to suggest that doxazosin may have beneficial effects on erectile function. Despite all the interest and controversy that surrounds the relative merits of subtype-selective agents, it is important not to lose sight of the main aim of α-blockade as recently described by Chapple; "from the clinical perspective the goal for pharmacological therapy for prostate disease is to produce a drug which is cost-effective, safe and has the greatest efficacy with the most beneficial adjunctive effects for the individual patient".[6]

Surgical management of benign prostatic obstruction

While there have been few recent innovations in the surgical management of BPH, our understanding of the therapies introduced over the past 3–4 years has been consolidated. Most of the research in this area has dealt with the delivery of various forms of energy (e.g. laser, ultrasound, radiofrequency, microwaves) to produce thermal damage, and thus tissue loss, within the prostate gland.

Recent evidence supports previous claims that some of the symptomatic improvement that follows these thermal treatments may be mediated by

Highlights in **Benign prostatic hyperplasia** 1997

WHAT'S IN ?

- Long-acting α_1-adrenoceptor antagonists
- Prophylactic medical treatment for acute urinary retention
- Holmium laser resection of the prostate

WHAT'S OUT ?

- Shorter-acting α_1-adrenoceptor antagonists
- Side-fire induced laser coagulation

local nerve destruction rather than prostatic debulking. For example, Zlotta and colleagues found that transurethral needle ablation (TUNA) resulted in complete loss of nerve fibres within the treated area.[7] These findings may help to explain the apparent paradox of significant subjective symptomatic improvement with minimal objective evidence of the relief of obstruction that is commonly reported in Phase III trials involving prostatic heat treatments.[8,9]

The histopathological response of the prostate to thermal injury has been investigated by Orihuela and colleagues.[10] They demonstrated that the re-epithelialization that follows laser irradiation takes 12 weeks to complete and results from the migration of proliferating epithelial cells from remaining acinar and ductal epithelium in a manner analogous to that seen in second-degree skin burns.

Most interest has centred on novel therapies that mimic TURP by providing immediate removal of tissue with less blood loss. A few studies have been published attesting to the safety and efficacy of both electrovaporization and holmium laser resection.

- Narayan reported satisfactory subjective and objective outcomes after electrovaporization of the prostate in 167 patients, but noted irritative voiding symptoms in 22.6% and urinary tract infections in 4.8%.[11]

- Chilton reported similar efficacy results following holmium laser resection in 873 patients and observed a low blood transfusion rate of 0.2%.[12]
- Patel demonstrated that the use of a computer-controlled constant power output radiofrequency generator allowed similar power settings to be used for both TURP and electrovaporization, and noted no adverse temperature rise in important structures located at the prostatic perimeter (i.e. external sphincter and neurovascular bundles).[13]

The evolution of laser use in the treatment of BPH continues following the slow demise of side-fire induced laser coagulation, and the continued growth of interstitial and contact techniques alongside the emergence of the holmium laser as a 'jack of all trades'. The results of updated randomized comparisons of these newer techniques with TURP are eagerly awaited.

Finally, the role of photodynamic therapy in both benign and malignant prostatic disease is being extensively investigated world-wide. The preliminary animal experiments with new photosensitizing agents are encouraging and suggest that the first human trials may be reported in the near future.[14]

References

1. Jacobsen S, Jacobsen D, Girman C et al. Natural history of prostatism; risk factors for acute urinary retention. J Urol 1997;158:481–7.

2. Andersen J, Curtis Nickel J, Marshall V, Schulman C, Boyle P. Finasteride significantly reduces acute urinary retention and need for surgery in patients with symptomatic benign prostatic hyperplasia. Urology 1997;49:839–45.

3. Kirby R, Pool J. Alpha adrenoceptor blockade in the treatment of benign prostatic hyperplasia: past, present and future. Br J Urol 1997;80:521–32.

4. Abrams P, Speakman M, Stott M, Arkell D, Pocock R. A dose-ranging study of the efficacy and safety of tamsulosin, the first prostate-selective α_{1A}-adrenoceptor antagonist, in patients with benign prostatic obstruction (symptomatic benign prostatic hyperplasia). Br J Urol 1997;80:587–96.

5. Lee E, Lee C. Clinical comparision of selective and non-selective α_{1A}-adrenoceptor antagonists in benign prostatic hyperplasia: studies on tamsulosin in a fixed dose and terazosin in increasing doses. Br J Urol 1997;80:606–11.

6. Chapple C. Editorial comment. Br J Urol 1997;79:904–6.

7. Zlotta A, Raviv G, Peny M-O, Noel J-C, Haot J, Schulman C. Possible mechanisms of action of transurethral needle ablation of the prostate on benign prostatic hyperplasia symptoms: a neurohistochemical study. *J Urol* 1997;157:894–9.

8. Mostafid A, Harrison N, Thomas P, Fletcher M. A prospective randomised trial of interstitial radiofrequency therapy versus transurethral resection for the treatment of benign prostatic hyperplasia. *Br J Urol* 1997;80:116–22.

9. Ahmed M, Bell T, Lawrence W, Ward J, Watson G. Transurethral microwave thermotherapy (Prostatron version 2.5) compared with transurethral resection of benign prostatic hyperplasia: a randomised, controlled, parallel study. *Br J Urol* 1997;79:181–5.

10. Orihuela E, Pow-Sang M, Motamedi M, Cowan D, Warren M. Mechanism of healing of the human prostatic urethra following thermal injury. *Urology* 1997;48:600–8.

11. Narayan P, Tewari A, Schalow E, Leidich R, Aboseif S, Cascione C. Transurethral evaporation of the prostate for treatment of benign prostatic hyperplasia: results in 168 patients with up to 12 months of follow-up. *J Urol* 1997;157:1309–12.

12. Chilton C, Gilling P, Fraundorfer M, Creswell M. The results of holmium laser resection of the prostate. *Br J Urol* 1997;79(S4):61.

13. Patel A, Fuchs G, Gutierrez-Aceves J, Ryan T. Prostate heating patterns comparing electrosurgical transurethral resection and vaporization: a prospective randomized study. *J Urol* 1997;157:169–72.

14. Shetty S, Peabody J, Beck E, Cerny J. Photodynamic therapy (PDT) for treating benign prostatic hyperplasia (BPH): a canine pilot study using liposomal benzoporphyin derivative (BPD). *Br J Urol* 1997;80(S2):192.

Prostate cancer

AR Zlotta and CC Schulman

Department of Urology, Erasme Hospital, University Clinics of Brussels, Belgium

Genetics of prostate cancer

HPC1 (for *Hereditary Prostate Cancer 1*), a specific gene that predisposes men to develop prostate cancer, has been located on chromosome 1. This gene was present in one third of members of families with known hereditary prostate cancer in North America and Sweden.[1,2] These studies provide the first evidence that specific genes for prostate cancer exist. Identification of such genes may provide new strategies for prevention, detection and treatment of this disease.

Epidemiology

Racial differences. The higher incidence of prostate cancer among black men has been confirmed.[3] Similarly, among men without histological evidence of prostate cancer, African-Americans have significantly higher PSA levels, age-specific PSA levels, and PSA densities.[4,5] Race-specific data are, therefore, needed to optimize PSA as a tumour marker in racial populations that are at high risk for prostate cancer.

Diet. Intake of essential fatty acids has been linked to the development and growth of prostate cancer.[6] Men whose diet was high in omega-3 fatty acid had a lower incidence of clinical prostate cancer. A positive association between intake of alpha-linolenic, palmitoleic and palmitic acid and risk of later prostate cancer was found in Norwegian men.[7]

A low fat diet may lead to a reduction in serum PSA without altering testosterone levels.[8] Further data are needed to determine the significance and mechanism of this effect, which may suggest chemopreventive strategies for prostate cancer.

Diagnosis

New biopsy techniques. The sextant biopsy technique has been used widely, and successfully, for diagnosing carcinoma of the prostate. However,

Highlights in **Prostate cancer** 1997

WHAT'S IN ?

Detection/diagnosis

- Genetics
- Free:total PSA

Treatment

- Radiotherapy and neoadjuvant hormonal treatment

WHAT'S NEW ?

Diagnosis

- PSA-TZ
- New biopsy techniques

Treatment

- 3D radiotherapy

WHAT'S OUT ?

Detection

- PSA velocity

Staging

- DNA ploidy

WHAT'S CONTROVERSIAL ?

Diagnosis and staging

- RT-PCR

Treatment

- Neoadjuvant hormonal treatment before radical prostatectomy
- Maximal androgen blockade

concern has arisen that the original sextant method may not include adequate sampling of the prostate. A prospective study of 512 patients showed that the standard sextant protocol leaves 15% of cancers undetected compared with results obtained from a more extensive biopsy procedure using 8 to 10 biopsies.[9] The '5 region prostate biopsy', which is a new method that takes sextant biopsies and additional biopsies in a systematic fashion, has been shown to be efficacious and superior to the sextant method of biopsy in the identification of prostate cancer at an early but significant stage.[10]

While the sensitivity increases when systematic and target sampling are combined, the clinical importance of cancers detected by multiple biopsies needs to be evaluated.

Serum markers

PSA testing intervals. For men with no cancer suspected on DRE, a PSA level of 4–5 ng/ml is an acceptable range for maintaining the detection of curable prostate cancer. These men should be monitored annually. When the initial PSA is less than 2.0 ng/ml, PSA testing should be carried out every 2 years, rather than on a yearly basis.[11] As 70% of a screened population between the ages of 50 and 70 years has a PSA level below 2.0 ng/ml, elimination of annual testing for these men could save considerable healthcare expenditure.

Free:total PSA. As further demonstrated by studies using either referred patients or patients included in screening programmes, use of the free:total PSA (F:T PSA) ratio may increase the specificity of serum PSA, without changing sensitivity, for prostate cancer detection in men with intermediate (4–10 ng/ml) PSA.[12–18] Most studies have found that, using F:T PSA, the number of unnecessary biopsies is decreased by 20–40%, while 95% of the cancers are detected.

Even in men with serum PSA concentrations of 2.6–4.0 ng/ml and normal DRE, Catalona *et al.* found that free PSA increased the specificity for prostate cancer prediction.[19]

Several studies have confirmed that, regardless of assay type, the proportion of free PSA increases with age.[20,21] Prostate size also significantly influences the level of free PSA in patients with prostate cancer.[16,18,21]

F:T PSA was only able to discriminate significantly between prostate cancer and BPH in men with a prostate volume of less than 40 cm^3.[16]

Percentage of free PSA does not help predict extracapsular disease in patients with clinically localized prostate cancer prior to radical prostatectomy.[15] However, levels of free PSA can predict cancer aggressiveness. This was demonstrated in a longitudinal study of 20 men diagnosed with adenocarcinoma of the prostate: frozen sera samples were available up to 18 years before the diagnosis of aggressive or non-aggressive prostate cancer was made.[22]

PSA density in the transition zone. Most PSA leakage from the prostate into the serum comes from the transition zone, and BPH arises almost exclusively from hyperplasia of the transition zone. As a result, transition-zone PSA density (PSA-TZ), which relates serum PSA to the volume of the transition zone (as determined by TRUS), has been suggested as a useful tool (and one that is significantly better than PSA density – PSAD – which relates serum PSA to the volume of the prostate) for enhancing the prediction of prostate cancer in men with serum PSA in the 4–10 ng/ml range. PSA-TZ thus minimizes unnecessary biopsies in men with benign disease.[23-26] Creasy *et al.*, in a study including 240 consecutive patients, found that PSA-TZ would have decreased the number of unnecessary biopsies by 22% while detecting 97% of cancers.[27] In another study, PSA-TZ spared 18% of unnecessary biopsies and detected 100% of the malignant lesions.[28]

Staging

Partin and coworkers have published their update on the well-known Partin's tables. This multi-institutional study included 4133 men who had undergone radical retropubic prostatectomy. Using updated nomograms, the authors found that PSA, TNM clinical stage and Gleason score on the prostate biopsy contributed significantly to the prediction of pathological stage of localized prostate cancer. In close to 75% of the time, the nomograms correctly predicted the probability of a pathological stage within a 10% error margin.[29]

Molecular techniques. The role of reverse transcriptase-polymerase chain reaction (RT-PCR) technology in the detection of extracapsular disease has been investigated by many groups, with conflicting results. Limiting factors in the detection of micrometastatic tumour cells by RT-PCR are:

- the transcription of tumour-associated or epithelial-specific genes from haematopoietic cells such as lymphocytes (!)
- expression deficiencies of the marker gene in micrometastatic tumour cells.[30]

Treatment of localized prostate cancer

Radical prostatectomy and predictive factors of outcome. Long-term results of radical prostatectomy in men with clinically localized prostate cancer have now been published. Analysing survival after radical prostatectomy in 3626 men from nine regions of the USA, Krongrad *et al.* found that older age and black race were independently associated with worse overall, but not disease-specific, survival. Estimates of 10-year disease-specific survival ranged from 75% to 97% for patients with well-differentiated and moderately differentiated cancers, and from 60% to 86% for patients with poorly differentiated cancers. Neither disease-specific nor overall survival varied by region, suggesting that disease-specific survival varied substantially by prostate cancer, but not patient, characteristics.[31]

In a multivariate analysis of 721 men with long-term follow-up, tumours with Gleason score 2–4 were almost all cured following radical prostatectomy, with 96% remaining progression-free over 10 years. In contrast, only 35% of patients with Gleason score 8–9 remained progression-free for the same period. For the majority of cases (i.e. those with intermediate Gleason scores), margin status did not provide further useful information about patients with capsular penetration, but prediction of their risk of progression was clearly enhanced by knowledge of pathological status.[32]

These studies offer the best currently available estimates of 10-year outcome of radical prostatectomy in men with clinically localized prostate cancer and may be useful in counselling patients with early malignancy.

Independent of the Gleason score, microvascular invasion might be a very important parameter to take into account as a predictor of bad prognosis after radical prostatectomy.[33,34]

Androgen withdrawal prior to or after radiation therapy. Neoadjuvant hormonal therapy has been shown to reduce both the volume of the irradiated adjacent tissues, which are thus spared, and the radiation dose. Adjuvant treatment with LHRH agonists, when started simultaneously with external irradiation, spectacularly improves local control and survival in patients with locally advanced prostate cancer. Indeed, in a randomized, prospective trial comparing external irradiation with external irradiation plus a LHRH agonist, 85% of surviving patients in the combined-treatment group were free from disease at 5 years, compared with 48% in the radiotherapy group ($p < 0.001$; median follow-up 45 months).[35]

In the Radiation Therapy Oncology Group (RTOG) trial, androgen suppression as an adjuvant to definitive radiotherapy was associated with a significant improvement in local control and freedom from disease progression. With a median follow-up time of 4.5 years, a significant improvement in survival was observed only in patients with tumours of Gleason score 8–10.[36]

Three-dimensional conformal radiation therapy uses computers to help pinpoint the tumour, so allowing the delivery of a much higher radiation dose to a very localized area without damaging the adjacent tissues.

Analysing the outcomes of treatment in 456 consecutive patients with prostate cancer treated with conformal three-dimensional radiation therapy, and defining biochemical failure as two consecutive rises in the PSA that equal or exceed 1.5 ng/ml, Hanks *et al.* found that the biochemical-failure-free (bNED) rate for all patients was 61% at 5 years and 57% at 7 years.[37] In the group with pretreatment PSA less than 10 ng/ml, the 5-year bNED rate for patients with localized disease (T1,2AB disease, Gleason score 6 or less) was 85%; for those with locally advanced disease (T2C,3), the 5-year bNED rate was 70%. In the group with pretreatment PSA of 20 ng/ml or above, patients with localized or locally advanced disease had 5-year bNED rates of 31% and 21%, respectively.

Brachytherapy involves placing radioactive material (temporary or permanent radioisotope seeds) directly into a malignancy. Because of the short range of this form of radiation, high doses may be delivered to a cancer, while the adjacent tissues are spared.

Currently, palladium-103 radioisotope is introduced into the prostate using a percutaneous transperineal approach. Results after this type of therapy for localized prostate cancer are interesting and deserve further attention.[38] Stone *et al.* found a positive biopsy rate of 21% in 75 patients with localized prostate cancer, followed for a minimum of 18 months after brachytherapy. Patients had received either iodine-125 (Gleason 6 or less) or palladium-103 (Gleason 7 and above) implants.[39]

Treatment of advanced prostate cancer

Maximal androgen blockade. Crawford *et al.*, in a multicentre prospective study of 1387 patients, found no difference in terms of survival or quality of life between patients receiving bilateral orchiectomy only, and those receiving orchiectomy plus flutamide.[40] Orchiectomy plus flutamide did, however, reduce PSA levels.

In contrast, a large double-blind trial on 457 patients randomized to receive nilutamide or placebo after orchiectomy, with 8.5 years follow-up, showed that combination therapy had significant benefits in terms of interval to progression and survival, compared with orchiectomy and placebo.[41]

Liarazole is a retinoic acid blocking agent developed as differentiation therapy for prostate cancer. It was demonstrated to promote the differentiation of cancer cells by increasing intratumoural levels of retinoic acid. Fradet *et al.* analysed the efficacy and safety of liarazole compared with cyproterone acetate in patients with advanced prostate cancer for whom first-line androgen ablative therapy had failed.[42] Of 321 patients, 160 were randomized to liarazole and 161 to cyproterone acetate. Liarazole conferred a 26% increase in survival benefit and a slight increase in survival time of 3.6 months. Time to progression was significantly longer in the liarazole-treated group, though it was only 1.2 months. Further studies are anticipated.

Gene therapy and immunological treatments

Future applications of gene therapy or immunological treatments for prostate cancer have been extensively studied. These new approaches will not necessarily replace surgical treatments, but might well be given in addition to current treatments. Briefly, many authors have, in the laboratory and in preliminary clinical studies, investigated the use of gene replacement, insertion of a suicide gene, and PSA gene regulation.

Immunological studies have used, for example, monoclonal antibodies directed against antigens expressed by prostatic epithelial cells, such as PROST 30.[43] In 41% of patients, PSA decreased by at least 20% and remained below pretreatment levels for 4–75+ weeks. In 23%, PSA decreased by at least 50% (50–66%) and remained below pretreatment levels for 8–75+ weeks. There were no side-effects related to the antibody treatment.

A recent Phase I clinical trial involved the administration of autologous dendritic cells pulsed with prostate-specific membrane antigen peptides to patients with advanced prostate cancer. Dendritic cells are called antigen professional carriers increasing antigen presentation and, therefore, enhancing the specific immune response. Responses in this initial Phase I trial were significant and of long duration.[44] Other forms of immunotherapy for prostate cancer may include prostatic acid phosphatase to induce destructive autoimmune prostatitis.[45]

References

1. Smith JR, Carpten J, Kallioniemi O *et al*. Major susceptibility locus for prostate cancer on chromosome 1 revealed by a genome-wide search. *Science* 1996;274: 1371–4.

2. Cooney KA, McCarthy JD, Lange E *et al*. Prostate cancer susceptibility locus on chromosome 1q: a confirmatory study. *J Natl Cancer Inst* 1997;89:955–9.

3. Smith DS, Bullock AD, Catalona WJ, Herschman JD. Racial differences in a prostate cancer screening study. *J Urol* 1996;156:1366–9.

4. Henderson RJ, Eastham JA, Culkin DJ *et al*. Prostate-specific antigen (PSA) and PSA density: racial differences in men without prostate cancer. *J Natl Cancer Inst* 1997;89:134–8.

5. Morgan TO, Jacobsen SJ, McCarthy WF, Jacobson DJ, McLeod DG, Moul JW. Age-specific reference ranges for serum prostate-specific antigen in black men. *N Engl J Med* 1996;335:304–10.

6. Pienta KJ, Goodson JA, Esper PS. Epidemiology of prostate cancer: molecular and environmental clues. *Urology* 1996;48:676–83.

7. Harvei S, Bjerve KS, Tretli S, Jellum E, Robsahm TE, Vatten L. Prediagnostic level of fatty acids in serum phospholipids: omega-3 and omega-6 fatty acids and the risk of prostate cancer. *Int J Cancer* 1997;71:545–51.

8. Fleshner NE, Schaeffer A, Shike M *et al*. Effects of a low fat dietary plan on serum prostate specific antigen levels in men with negative prostate needle biopsies: preliminary results. *J Urol* 1997;157(Suppl):A430.

9. Norberg M, Egevad L, Holmberg L, Sparen P, Norlen BJ, Busch C. The sextant protocol for ultrasound-guided core biopsies of the prostate underestimates the presence of cancer. *Urology* 1997;50:562–6.

10. Eskew LA, Bare RL, McCullough DL. Systematic 5 region prostate biopsy is superior to sextant method for diagnosing carcinoma of the prostate. *J Urol* 1997;157:199–202.

11. Carter HB, Epstein JI, Chan DW, Fozard JL, Pearson JD. Recommended prostate-specific antigen testing intervals for the detection of curable prostate cancer. *JAMA* 1997;277:1456–60.

12. Abrahamsson P-A, Lilja H, Oesterling JE. Molecular forms of serum prostate-specific antigen. *Urol Clin N Am* 1997;24:353–65.

13. Akdas A, Cevik I, Tarcan T, Turkeri L, Dalaman G, Emerk K. The role of free prostate-specific antigen in the diagnosis of prostate cancer. *Br J Urol* 1997;79:920–3.

14. Bangma CH, Rietbergen JB, Kranse R, Blijenberg BG, Petterson K, Schroder FH. The free-to-total prostate specific antigen ratio improves the specificity of prostate specific antigen in screening for prostate cancer in the general population. *J Urol* 1997;157:2191–6.

15. Morote J, Raventos CX, Lorente JA *et al.* Measurement of free PSA in the diagnosis and staging of prostate cancer. *Int J Cancer* 1997;71:756–9.

16. Stephan C, Lein M, Jung K, Schnorr D, Loening SA. The influence of prostate volume on the ratio of free to total prostate specific antigen in serum of patients with prostate carcinoma and benign prostate hyperplasia. *Cancer* 1997;79:104–9.

17. Egawa S, Soh S, Ohori M *et al.* The ratio of free to total serum prostate specific antigen and its use in differential diagnosis of prostate carcinoma in Japan. *Cancer* 1997;79:90–8.

18. Catalona WJ, Ornstein DK, Humphrey PA, Smith DS. Factors affecting the percentage of free serum prostate specific antigen levels in men without clinically detectable prostate cancer. *J Urol* 1997;157(Suppl):A433.

19. Catalona WJ, Smith DS, Ornstein DK. Prostate cancer detection in men with serum PSA concentrations of 2.6 to 4.0 ng/ml and benign prostate examination. Enhancement of specificity with free PSA measurements. *JAMA* 1997;277:1452–5.

20. Vashi AR, Wojno KJ, Vessella RL *et al.* Percent free PSA correlates directly with patient age. J Urol 1997;157(Suppl):A432.

21. Partin AW, Catalona WJ, Southwick PC, Subong EN, Gasior GH, Chan DW. Analysis of percent free prostate-specific antigen (PSA) for prostate cancer detection: influence of total PSA, prostate volume, and age. *Urology* 1996;48(Suppl):55–61.

22. Carter HB, Partin AW, Chan DW, Luderer A, Pearson JD. Percentage of free PSA in sera predicts cancer aggressiveness: a longitudinal analysis. *J Urol* 1997;157(Suppl):A444.

23. Zlotta AR, Djavan B, Marberger M, Schulman CC. Prostate specific antigen density of the transition zone: a new effective parameter for prostate cancer prediction. *J Urol* 1997;157:1315–21.

24. Kurita Y, Ushiyama T, Suzuki K, Fujita K, Kawabe K. PSA value adjusted for the transition zone volume in the diagnosis of prostate cancer. *Int J Urol* 1996;3:367–72.

25. Maeda H, Ishitoya S, Maekawa Y *et al.* Prostate specific antigen density of the transition zone in the detection of prostate cancer. *J Urol* 1997;157(Suppl): A219.

26. Kiewert A, Loch T, Küppers F, Schmidt S, Stöckle M. Correlation of prostate specific antigen (PSA) serum levels with prostatic glandular zone volumes. *J Urol* 1997;157(Suppl):A453.

27. Creasy T, Lesna M, Rundle D, Bramble J, Morley R. Central gland PSA density – a more sensitive tool for the diagnosis of carcinoma of the prostate. *J Urol* 1997;157(Suppl):A209.

28. Horninger W, Reissigl A, Klockler H, Höltl L, Fink K, Bartsch G. Improvement of early detection of prostate cancer by using PSA-transitional zone density (PSA-TZ density) and percent free PSA in addition to total PSA levels. *J Urol* 1997;157(Suppl):A454.

29. Partin AW, Kattan MW, Subong EN *et al.* Combination of prostate specific antigen, clinical stage, and Gleason score to predict pathological stage of localized prostate cancer. A multi-institutional update. *JAMA* 1997;277:1445–51.

30. Zippelius A, Kufer P, Honols G *et al.* Limitations of reverse-transcriptase polymerase chain reaction analyses for detection of micrometastatic epithelial cells in bone marrow. *J Clin Oncol* 1997;15:2701–8.

31. Krongrad A, Lai H, Lai S. Survival after radical prostatectomy. *JAMA* 1997;278:44–6.

32. Epstein JI, Partin AW, Sauvageot J, Walsh PC. Prediction of progression following radical prostatectomy: a multivariate analysis of 721 men with long-term follow-up. *Amer J Surg Path* 1996;20:286–92.

33. van den Ouden D, Kranse R, Hop WC, Schröder FH. Microvascular invasion in relation to tumor control in patients with prostate cancer treated by radical prostatectomy. *J Urol* 1997;157(Suppl):A1154.

34. Bettencourt MC, Sesterhenn I, Connelly R, Bauer J, Moul J. Angiogenesis is a prognostic marker of prostate cancer recurrence after radical prostatectomy. *J Urol* 1997;157(Suppl): A1156.

35. Bolla M, Gonzalez D, Warde P *et al.* Improved survival in patients with locally advanced prostate cancer treated with radiotherapy and goserelin. *N Engl J Med* 1997;337:295–300.

36. Pilepich MV, Caplan R, Byhardt RW *et al.* Phase III trial of androgen suppression using goserelin in unfavorable-prognosis carcinoma of the prostate treated with definitive radiotherapy: report of Radiation Therapy Oncology Group Protocol 85-31. *J Clin Oncol* 1997;15:1013–21.

37. Hanks GE, Hanlon AL, Schultheiss TE *et al.* Conformal external beam treatment of prostate cancer. *Urology* 1997;50:87–92.

38. Blasko JC, Ragde H, Luse RW, Sylvester JE, Cavanagh W, Grimm PD. Should brachytherapy be considered a therapeutic option in localized prostate cancer? *Urol Clin North Am* 1996;23: 633–50.

39. Stone N, Stock R, Unger P. Prostate biopsy results following brachytherapy for localized prostate cancer: an analysis of variables influencing outcomes. *J Urol* 1997;157(Suppl):A1632.

40. Crawford ED, Eisenberger MA, McLeod DG, Wilding G, Blumenstein BA. Comparison of bilateral orchiectomy with or without flutamide for the treatment of patients (PTS) with stage D2, adenocarcinoma of the prostate (CaP): Results of NCI intergroup study 0105 (SWOG and ECOG). *J Urol* 1997;157(Suppl):A1311.

41. Dijkman GA, Janknegt RA, De Reijke TM, Debruyne FM. Long-term efficacy and safety of nilutamide plus castration in advanced prostate cancer, and the significance of early prostate specific antigen normalization. International Anandron Study Group. *J Urol* 1996;158:160.

42. Fradet Y, Trachtenberg J. Liazal (liarazole) vs cyproterone acetate in advanced prostate cancer: results of a randomized phase III trial. *J Urol* 1997;157(Suppl):A1305.

43. Shemtov M, Bander NH. Phase I/II trial of monoclonal antibody PROST 30 in advanced prostate cancer. *J Urol* 1997;157(Suppl):A1256.

44. Tjoa BA, Erickson SJ, Bowes VA *et al.* Follow-up evaluation of prostate cancer patients infused with autologous dendritic pulsed with PSMA peptides. *Prostate* 1997;32:272–8.

45. Fong L, Ruegg CL, Brockstedt D, Engleman EG, Laus R. Induction of tissue-specific autoimmune prostatitis with prostatic acid phosphatase immunization: implications for immunotherapy of prostate cancer. *J Immunol* 1997;159:3113–17.

Bladder cancer

MF Sarosdy

Division of Urology, University of Texas Health Science Center, San Antonio, Texas, USA

Diagnostic tests

The development and optimization of rapid, point of care, diagnostic tests for bladder cancer is continuing. The BTA *stat* test for bladder tumour antigen (BTA), and the AuraTek FDP test for fibrin/fibrinogen degradation products, are both immunoassay systems that use unbuffered urine as the test sample.

In a large, retrospective, comparative analysis using frozen urine from a previous multicentre study, Sarosdy *et al.* reported an overall BTA *stat* sensitivity of 67% in 220 patients with histologically confirmed bladder cancer.[1] The sensitivity of the original BTA test on a large portion of specimens had been 44%, while the BTA *stat* test detected 58% and voided cytology detected 23%. Specificity of the BTA *stat* test in healthy volunteers was 95%.

In 192 patients with a history of bladder cancer, Schmetter *et al.* compared the AuraTek FDP with urinary cytology or haemoglobin dipstick.[2] The AuraTek FDP detected disease in 68% of patients, cytology detected 34%, and haemoglobin dipstick detected 41%. Specificity of the AuraTek FDP was 96% for healthy subjects, 86% in patients with urological disease other than bladder cancer, and 80% in patients with a history of bladder cancer but no tumour found at cystoscopy.

The role of these new diagnostic tests in practice remains to be determined by prospective trials. The need for diagnostic tests other than cystoscopy and cytology is further supported by the report of Grégoire *et al.*[3] Comparing voided cytology, bladder wash cytology and flow cytometry in 166 patients followed for bladder cancer recurrence, they found that both flow cytometry and cytology performed on bladder wash samples added little information to that obtained from voided urine cytology.

Prognostic markers

A number of prognostic markers continue to be evaluated. Chief among these is the *p53* tumour suppressor gene. Unfortunately, of patients whose tumours stain positively for *p53*, approximately half later progress to muscle invasion and half do not. Raitanen *et al.* reported that 17 of 29 (59%) Ta or T1 patients eventually progressed to a stage higher than T2 within 4 years, but only 5 of the 17 (29%) were initially *p53*-positive.[4] Similarly, Burkhard *et al.* found that among 46 superficial tumours, 27 (75%) of 36 *p53*-positive tumours did not progress to higher stage or metastatic disease.[5]

That a single prognostic marker may not be adequate to support treatment decisions, such as early cystectomy, is further supported by an updated report by Cordon-Cardo *et al.*[6] This details the Memorial experience in 59 patients with superficial transitional cell carcinoma (TCC) studied for alterations in *p53* and *RB* tumour suppressor genes. Patients with an alteration in either gene (shown by immunohistochemical staining) demonstrated increased stage progression compared with non-altered phenotypes. Nine patients with alterations in both *p53* and *RB* had an even higher rate of progression, and lower survival. Other tumour-related antigens (e.g. 486p, 19A211, M344) were present in histologically normal mucosa in locations away from tumours in patients with superficial disease.[7] Whether such early tumour-related changes suggest a need for early cystectomy or early intervention with intravesical immunotherapy remains to be determined.

Enthusiasm for 'aggressive therapy', including cystectomy, for patients with initial superficial tumours that are *p53*-positive should be tempered by reports that such status does not predict poor response to BCG therapy. Ick *et al.* reported that 21 of 23 cases (91%) of carcinoma *in situ* (CIS) were *p53*-positive, including 10 of 12 who subsequently received BCG.[8] Only four *p53*-positive patients demonstrated CIS after BCG, indicating that 60% responded to BCG. Their conclusion was that *p53* staining after BCG therapy was more helpful when deciding on the treatment course. Similarly, Ovesen *et al.* reported that intravesical BCG resulted in *p53*-negative staining in 73% of patients (n = 26) who were *p53*-positive prior to BCG therapy.[9] Also, progression related to *p53*-positivity after, not before, treatment.

Intravesical adjuvant therapy

Chemotherapy. Reports from randomized, prospective, controlled trials

Highlights in **Bladder cancer** *1997*

WHAT'S IN ?

- New, simpler diagnostic tests – BTA *stat*, AuraTek FDP
- Intravesical chemotherapy for recurrent, low-risk papillary tumours
- Maintenance BCG for high-risk disease, such as T1 or CIS, with liberal use of INH to decrease toxicity
- Orthotopic bladder replacement, even in women
- A search for more effective anti-cancer drugs for systemic disease

WHAT'S OUT ?

- *p53* as a single, stand-alone test for decision-making
- Frozen-section examination of ureteral margins at cystectomy
- MVAC as a standard first-line chemotherapy regimen

continue to demonstrate the efficacy of intravesical chemotherapy with respect to prevention of recurrence. Kurth *et al.* reported the results of a large, prospective, European Organization for Research and Treatment of Cancer (EORTC) trial of 443 patients with Ta or T1 lesions, with or without CIS, receiving transurethral resection (TUR) alone, or TUR plus either doxorubicin, 50 mg, or ethoglucid, 1.13 g, weekly for 1 month, then monthly for 1 year.[10] Time to first recurrence was significantly prolonged by both drugs, compared with TUR alone.

Ali-El-Dein *et al.* reported a prospective trial in which 253 patients with Ta or T1 tumours received TUR only or TUR followed by one of three regimens: epirubicin, 50 mg; epirubicin, 80 mg; or doxorubicin, 50 mg; weekly for 8 weeks, then monthly for 1 year.[11] Recurrence (%) and rates of recurrence/100 patient months, were markedly (and significantly) lower for all three chemotherapy groups compared with the TUR group. Furthermore, recurrence in both epirubicin groups was significantly lower than in the doxorubicin group. The higher dose of epirubicin also fared better than the lower dose. In neither the EORTC nor the Egyptian study did chemotherapy decrease progression to muscle disease. This reinforces the suggestion that chemotherapy may be appropriate for patients with frequent recurrences of tumours deemed to be at low risk of progression.

Immunotherapy. Two reports of clinical relevance, from the American Urological Association Meeting in New Orleans, Louisiana, should be noted, even though they are not yet published. The long-awaited final analysis of the Southwest Oncology Group (SWOG) trial of intravesical BCG for 6 weeks versus relatively intense maintenance therapy for 3 years was reported.[12] This large, randomized, prospective trial showed a significant reduction in untoward events (i.e. recurrence, progression, death) in the maintenance therapy group. Median time to recurrence was doubled. This benefit was seen despite reduction in the intended maintenance due to toxicity in a large number of patients.

Colleen *et al.* reported the results of a large, prospective trial of isoniazid (INH), which showed that INH, 300 mg given on 3 consecutive days around BCG-administration, reduced BCG-associated toxicity.[13] This does not mean that all patients treated with BCG should receive INH, but that the urologist should be comfortable initiating INH for the patient with significant symptoms not resolving within 12–24 hours of treatment.

Another issue is whether or not repeat BCG should be administered to patients who initially respond, but suffer a tumour recurrence. In a small but meaningful study, Bui and Schellhammer reported that, of 11 such patients, 9 (82%) achieved a second complete response, with 5 of those remaining tumour free for a median follow-up of 87 months (range 64–110).[14]

Cystectomy and urinary diversion

Some issues surrounding cystectomy and urinary diversion remain unsettled, including the timing of cystectomy for high-risk superficial disease, and the roles of neoadjuvant or adjuvant chemotherapy. One approach receiving particular attention is orthotopic lower tract reconstruction with urethra-sparing in women. Stein *et al.* reported satisfactory experience in 34 women, aged 31 to 86 years old (median age 67 years), with Koch neobladders.[15] Complete day- and night-time continence was reported in 88% and 82% of patients respectively, with only 15% requiring intermittent catheterization. Very similar results using ileal neobladders were reported by Stenzl *et al.*;[16] of the 30 patients followed, only 4% required self-catheterization.

The cost of care for the cystectomy patient is receiving more attention. Golden and Ratliff reported the development of a multidisciplinary clinical pathway to serve as a guide for radical cystectomy.[17] The implementation of this pathway focuses attention on efforts directed at improved clinical outcome, and reduced complications and cost. Two other studies have also indicated that frozen section analysis for ureteral margin at the time of cystectomy is unlikely to have any impact on clinical outcome, and the cost and time spent in pursuit of this may not be reasonable. Silver *et al.* reported that, in 401 patients undergoing cystectomy, concomitant ureteral CIS was uncommon;[18] frozen section failed to detect it in 5 of 30 patients in whom it was present. Similarly, Solsona and colleagues in Valencia reported an association of upper tract CIS with bladder tumour *in situ*, but that upper tract involvement alone had no impact on survival.[19]

Advanced/metastatic TCC

Patients still present with, or develop advanced disease after cystectomy. It is clear that methotrexate plus vinblastine plus doxorubicin plus cisplatin (MVAC) and other regimens developed in the 1980s are not sufficient for the majority of patients. Stadler *et al.* provided a timely review of several drugs including paclitaxel and gemcitabine.[20] Response rates of up to 33% in Phase II trials were reported with paclitaxel plus gemcitabine, supporting the need for further investigation of these and other new agents in combination.

References

1. Sarosdy MF, Hudson MA, Ellis WJ *et al.* Improved detection of recurrent bladder cancer using the Bard® BTA *stat*™ Test. *Urology* 1997;In press.

2. Schmetter BS, Habicht KK, Lamm DL *et al.* A multicenter trial evaluation of the fibrin/fibrinogen degradation products test for detection and monitoring of bladder cancer. *J Urol* 1997;158:801–5.

3. Grégoire M, Fradet Y, Meyers F *et al.* Diagnostic accuracy of urinary cytology, and deoxyribonucleic acid flow cytometry and cytology on bladder washings during followup for bladder tumours. *J Urol* 1997;157:1660–4.

4. Raitanen M-P, Tammela LJ, Kallioinen M, Isola J. P53 accumulation, deoxyribonucleic acid ploidy and progression of bladder cancer. *J Urol* 1997;157:1250–3.

5. Burkhardt FC, Markwalder R, Thalmann GN, Studer UE. Immunohistochemical determination of *p53* overexpression. An easy and readily available method to identify progression in superficial bladder cancer? *Urol Res* 1997;25:S31–5.

6. Cordon-Cardo C, Zhang ZF, Dalbagni G *et al.* Cooperative effects of *p53* and *pRB* alterations in primary superficial bladder tumours. *Cancer Res* 1997;57:1217–21.

7. Lee E, Schwaibold H, Fradet Y, Huland E, Huland H. Tumor-associated antigens in normal mucosa of patients with superficial transitional cell carcinoma of the bladder. *J Urol* 1997;157:1070–3.

8. Ick K, Schultz M, Stout P, Fan K. Significance of *p53* overexpression in urinary bladder transitional cell carcinoma *in situ* before and after Bacillus Calmette-Guerin treatment. *Urology* 1997;49:541–7.

9. Ovesen H, Horn T, Steven K. Long-term efficacy of intravesical Bacillus Calmette-Guerin for carcinoma *in situ*: relationship of progression to histological response and *p53* nuclear accumulation. *J Urol* 1997;157:1655–9.

10. Kurth K, Tunn U, Ay R *et al.* Adjuvant chemotherapy for superficial transitional cell bladder carcinoma: long-term results of a European Organization for Research and Treatment of Cancer randomized trial comparing doxorubicin, ethoglucid and transurethral resection alone. *J Urol* 1997;158:378–84.

11. Ali-El-Dein B, El-Baz M, Aly ANM *et al.* Intravesical epirubicin versus doxorubicin for superficial bladder tumours (stages pTa and pT1): a randomized prospective study. *J Urol* 1997;158:68–74.

12. Lamm DL, Blumenstein B, Sarosdy MF, Grossman HB, Crawford ED. Significant long-term patient benefit with BCG maintenance therapy: a Southwest Oncology Group study. *J Urol* 1997;157: 213A.

13. Colleen S, Elfving P, Khalifa M *et al.* The impact of concomitant isoniazid (INH) administration on side-effects, complications and anti-tumour effect of Bacillus Calmette-Guerin (BCG). *J Urol* 1997;157:161.

14. Bui TT, Schellhammer PF. Additional Bacillus Calmette-Guerin therapy for recurrent transitional cell carcinoma after an initial complete response. *Urology* 1997;49:687–91.

15. Stein JP, Grossfeld GD, Freeman JA *et al.* Orthotopic lower urinary tract reconstruction in women using the Koch ileal neobladder: updated experience in 34 patients. *J Urol* 1997;158:400–5.

16. Stenzl A, Colleselli K, Bartsch G. Update of urethra-sparing approaches in cystectomy in women. *World J Urol* 1997;15:134–8.

17. Golden TM, Ratliff C. Development and implementation of a clinical pathway for radical cystectomy and urinary system reconstruction. *J Wound Ostomy Continence Nurs* 1997;24:72–8.

18. Silver DA, Stroumbakis N, Russo P *et al*. Ureteral carcinoma *in situ* at radical cystectomy: does the margin matter? *J Urol* 1997;158:768–71.

19. Solsona E, Iborra I, Ricos JV *et al*. Upper urinary tract involvement in patients with bladder carcinoma *in situ* (Tis): its impact on management. *Urology* 1997;49:347–52.

20. Stadler WM, Kuzel TM, Raghavan D *et al*. Metastatic bladder cancer: advances in treatment. *Eur J Cancer* 1997;33:S23–6.

Andrology

JP Mulhall and I Goldstein

Departments of Urology, Loyola University Medical Center, Stritch School of Medicine, Loyola University, Chicago, and Boston Medical Center, Boston University School of Medicine, Boston, USA

Exciting developments in the non-invasive management of erectile dysfunction (ED) have once again been in the forefront in the field of andrology. Hand-in-hand with these innovations, a number of well established therapeutic modalities – inflatable penile prostheses and vasal reconstructive surgery following vasectomy – have received confirmation of their place in the andrologist's armamentarium.

Oral therapy in erectile dysfunction

The trend over recent years in the management of ED has been towards the development and application of minimally invasive modalities. As a result, the introduction of the first oral medications specifically designed for the treatment of impotent men is now on the horizon. The development of such agents is the direct result of a more complete understanding of the cellular and biochemical mechanisms involved in penile erection. Three agents are currently either undergoing trials or FDA investigation.

Sildenafil is a selective and competitive type V phosphodiesterase (PDE) inhibitor, which promotes accumulation of cyclic guanosine monophosphate (cGMP) within the smooth muscle cell.[1] This accumulation results in the sequestration of calcium in the endoplasmic reticulum and also its efflux from the cell, leading to a reduction in available intracellular calcium. This, in turn, causes smooth muscle relaxation, which results in penile erection.[2] In contrast to other agents, which have previously been used empirically, sildenafil appears to act specifically on corporal smooth muscle as type V PDE appears to be confined to erectile tissue.[1]

Sildenafil, 25, 50 or 100 mg, is administered 1 hour before sexual activity and, at higher doses of 50–100 mg, has improved erectile function in up to 77% of men.[3] Side-effects appear to be minimal, but include headache and

Highlights in **Andrology** 1997

WHAT'S IN ?

- Digoxin for idiopathic priapism
- Oral agents in impotence treatment
- Inflatable penile prostheses
- Vasectomy reversal surgery

WHAT'S OUT ?

- Malleable penile prostheses
- Testosterone administration

blurred vision. Sildenafil is awaiting FDA approval and is not licensed in the UK at time of press.

Apomorphine has direct central D_2-receptor agonist activity.[4] Morales and associates have recently developed a sublingual formulation that appears to be effective in many patients with minimal vasculogenic impotence.[4] In a carefully selected group of patients with psychogenic impotence, 8 of 12 patients (67%) receiving apomorphine experienced durable erections.[4]

Apomorphine is administered sublingually 20–40 minutes before sexual activity. It does, however, have a number of adverse effects, including persistent yawning, nausea, vomiting and hypotension.[4] Phase III trials are currently underway to evaluate the efficacy of apomorphine in the treatment of men with impotence of uncertain organic aetiology.

Phentolamine. Oral administration of the non-selective antagonist, phentolamine, has been shown to result in erection.[5] It has also been shown to have some anti-serotonin activity and a direct non-specific relaxant effect on blood vessels. Zorgniotti investigated the efficacy of phentolamine, 50 mg, in patients with psychogenic and mild arteriogenic ED and found that it produced a functional erection in 42% of patients.[6] These results were confirmed in a non-randomized, non-placebo controlled, multicentre trial in which patients received phentolamine, 20–40 mg, impregnated on a strip of filter paper applied to buccal mucosa 15 minutes before coitus.[7] In this study, 32% of patients obtained an erection suitable for intercourse versus 13% in the placebo group.

Inflatable penile prostheses

In those men in whom vasoactive therapy fails or who find it an undesirable form of therapy, the insertion of a penile prosthesis may be considered. The inflatable version of this device has recently been demonstrated to have a mechanical malfunction and infection rate as low as that of the semi-rigid or malleable devices.[8] Furthermore, these devices have been shown to have acceptable longevity, with a predicted re-operation rate of 15% at 10 years based on Kaplan-Meier analysis. While malleable implants have received acceptance among urological surgeons because of their ease of insertion, the inflatable prosthesis remains the device of choice because of the current similarity in complication rates, the development of devices that are easier to implant and the improved patient satisfaction rates.

With the advent of the two-piece inflatable device, even those surgeons who only occasionally carry out such implants should feel comfortable using them. While the two-piece implant does not have the same rigidity or girth profile of its three-piece counterpart, it is of value following radical cystectomy in men who have peritonealization of the space of Retzius, in whom there is a risk of viscus perforation with the use of a reservoir. Other men who may benefit from implantation of a two-piece device include those who have undergone radical prostatectomy and those who have had bilateral inguinal hernia surgery.

Digoxin for idiopathic priapism

Although the most common cause of priapism in adult men is the use of intracavernosal pharmacological agents, there are some men who develop prolonged erections for no overt aetiological reason and suffer from recurrent idiopathic priapism. This condition is poorly understood, but most probably results from an imbalance between erectogenic and erectolytic mechanisms, which results in unregulated smooth muscle relaxation unrelated to sexual stimulation, leading to an uncontrolled prolonged erection.

The therapeutic options currently available have failed to manage the recurrent nature of this problem adequately. Only one small study, which was non-randomized and uncontrolled, has demonstrated that the periodic intramuscular administration of luteinizing hormone releasing hormone (LHRH) agonists ameliorates this condition.[9] As with all LHRH agonist therapy, concerns exist regarding the effect of this therapy on the patient's libido. Given the generally young age of this patient population, any treatment that interferes with sexual interest will inevitably result in reduced patient acceptance and compliance.

Digoxin is a powerful inotropic agent used extensively in the management of the failing myocardium. It is a Na^+K^+-ATPase inhibitor, which increases the available intracellular calcium and thus promotes smooth muscle contraction.[10] While this aids the failing heart, in the penis, it leads to a failure to develop erection or detumescence of an erection. *In vitro*, digoxin contracts corporal smooth muscle forcibly and, *in vivo*, has been shown to reduce the number and rigidity of nocturnal erections in young healthy male volunteers by Rigiscan® analysis.[11] Furthermore, data from multiple centres supports the use of digoxin in the management of idiopathic priapism. Following metabolic and cardiac clearance, digoxin, 1 g, is administered over a 24-hour period and the dose titrated to maintain a therapeutic serum level. Thus far, this approach has been successful and awaits validation in a randomized, placebo-controlled trial.

Vasal reconstructive surgery

Following the ground-breaking work of the vasectomy reversal study group in 1990,[12] vasal reconstruction was firmly established as a management strategy for men who had undergone a vasectomy and who wished to have more children. This group, in an analysis of over 1200 patients who underwent microscopic vasectomy reversal demonstrated patency rates as high as 97% in men 3 years post-vasectomy and 70% in men 15 years post-vasectomy. Pregnancy rates of 75% and 30%, respectively, were reported following the same postoperative intervals.

Since the introduction of advanced reproductive technologies, such as intracytoplasmic sperm injection (ICSI), the role of vasectomy reversal has been called into question. Some authorities have suggested that sperm aspiration, whether epididymal or testicular in origin, should be used in conjunction with ICSI. The rationale behind this is that expensive surgery can be avoided, while at the same time achieving a pregnancy rate similar to that of ICSI in men more than 10 years post-vasectomy. As a result, some centres are promoting percutaneous sperm retrieval from either the epididymis (PESA) or testis (TESA). The drive behind this philosophy has, however, emanated from our colleagues working in the field of reproductive endocrinology/ gynaecology and, unfortunately, has ignored a number of issues.

Comparison of risk. Most urologists, particularly those trained in microsurgical techniques perform vasal reconstruction as an out-patient procedure with minimal anaesthesia; local anaesthesia to the scrotum combined with intravenous sedation is generally used. The procedure is well tolerated by patients, most of whom return to work within a few days. Thus, vasectomy reversal surgery should not be looked upon as a highly invasive procedure. In contrast, sperm aspirated from the epididymis or testis must be used in conjunction with ICSI and cannot be used in other techniques, such as intrauterine insemination or even conventional *in vitro* fertilization with any success. Thus, while the man may be spared a minor surgery, his female partner is exposed to the pharmacological manipulation that is required to induce ovulation prior to oocyte harvesting.

Ovulation induction usually comprises intramuscular LHRH agonists initially, followed by daily intramuscular or subcutaneous gonadotrophins. During this process, blood samples must be taken regularly to monitor oestradiol levels to assess the ovarian response, and regular transvaginal ultrasound examinations must be performed to assess the size of the developing oocytes. The eggs are then harvested transvaginally by needle aspiration prior to intracytoplasmic implantation of the sperm. In addition, ovarian stimulation is associated with a 5% incidence of hyperstimulation, which is a potentially serious complication.[13] Thus, it can readily be seen that, while ICSI may avoid surgery in the man, it is a far more complex option than vasal reconstruction that exposes the female partner to greater risks than would ever have been the case for the man.

Pregnancy rate. Epididymal or testicular sperm combined with ICSI achieves pregnancy in less than 40% of cases, even in the most experienced of hands.[14] Vasectomy reversal, however, achieves better pregnancy rates provided that it is performed less than 15 years after the original vasectomy and, even after

15 years, the pregnancy rate is similar to ICSI. Surgery also enables conception to occur naturally.

One of the drawbacks of surgery, however, is that it may take up to 9 months to determine whether sperm have returned to the ejaculate.[15] If the man's partner is over 38 years of age, time may be a major issue (oocyte viability may be poor and may deteriorate even further over a 6–9 month period) and, therefore, a more immediate solution, such as sperm aspiration and ICSI, may be preferable. Thus, it is incumbent on the clinician to ensure that the couple are given a fair and honest appraisal of the options to enable them to make an informed decision with which they are comfortable.

Cost-effectiveness. In terms of cost-effectiveness, vasectomy reversal is clearly superior to sperm aspiration and ICSI. The cost of sperm aspiration and ICSI is US$80,000/live birth compared with US$30,000/live birth following vasal reconstruction;[16] these costs take into account surgical costs as well as the cost of complications of therapy, including the multiple gestation associated with ICSI. Furthermore, it has recently been shown that, even in men who have already undergone vasectomy reversal, secondary vasal surgery is more cost-effective than sperm aspiration and ICSI.[17] Thus, in most men, vasectomy reversal performed by a trained microsurgeon is superior to sperm aspiration and ICSI in terms of cost-effectiveness, therapeutic outcome and safety profile.

Testosterone therapy for erectile dysfunction

Testosterone supplementation is one of the most commonly prescribed and mis-prescribed therapies for ED. What constitutes an adequate endocrine evaluation of an impotent man remains an unresolved issue. In order to put the role of endocrine evaluation into perspective, however, it must be appreciated that only a small proportion (< 5%) of men with impotence suffer from hypogonadism.[18]

If total serum testosterone level is low, the free testosterone level should be checked. Often, a low total serum testosterone level is an indication of elevated levels of sex-hormone-binding globulin and the free testosterone level is normal. If both the total and free testosterone levels are low, a state of chemical hypogonadism exists, and patients should be counselled regarding the risks and benefits of testosterone administration. There are no current data to support the use of supplemental androgens, such as testosterone or dehydroepiandrosterone, to induce supra-physiological serum levels for the treatment of erectile dysfunction. Furthermore, it has been demonstrated that, in hypogonadal men with impotence, administration of testosterone alone results in improvement of erection in only approximately 60% of patients.[19] The reason for this is multifactorial. Androgens are facilitators of erection and their absence does not necessarily preclude good erectile function. Furthermore, there are some hypogonadal men in whom ED is more dependent on vascular risk factors (e.g. diabetes, hypertension, hypercholesterolaemia, smoking) than low testosterone levels. In this population, testosterone administration will fail to improve ED.

Testosterone administration has been implicated in the development of BPH, acceleration of the growth of any pre-existing prostatic carcinoma, and elevation of serum lipid levels and the haematocrit. Testosterone should, therefore, only be prescribed once the patient has been fully informed of the pros and cons of therapy. Initially, testosterone is usually administered transdermally. If there is a problem with this route, it is given intramuscularly. Oral administration is avoided, because of the potential for liver damage. Therapy is instituted for a finite period of time and the patient's response carefully monitored. If no improvement in erectile function occurs, testosterone is generally withdrawn.

Thus, the role for testosterone administration in the management of the patient with ED is limited. Patients with documented hypogonadism should be counselled regarding the risks and benefits of therapy, and careful monitoring of patient response must be implemented.

References

1. Boolell M, Allen MJ, Ballard SA *et al.* Sildenafil: an orally active type 5 cyclic GMP-specific phosphodiesterase inhibitor for the treatment of penile erectile dysfunction. *Int J Impotence Res* 1996;8:47–52.

2. Porst H. The rationale for prostaglandin E1 in erectile failure: a survey of worldwide experience. *J Urol* 1996;55:802–15.

3. Lue TF. A study of sildenafil: a new oral agent for the treatment of male erectile dysfunction. *J Urol* 1997:157:181(Abstract 701).

4. Morales A, Heaton JP, Johnston B, Adams M. Oral and topical treatment of erectile dysfunction: present and future. *Urol Clin N Am* 1995;22:879–86.

5. Gwinup G. Oral phentolamine in non-specific erectile insufficiency. *Ann Intern Med* 1988;109:162–3.

6. Zorgniotti AW. 'On demand' oral drug for erection on impotent men. *J Urol* 1993;147:308(Abstract).

7. Wagner G, Lacy S, Lewis R. Buccal phentolamine: a pilot trial for male erectile dysfunction at three separate clinics. *Int J Impot Res* 1994;6(Suppl 1):D78.

8. Goldstein I, Newman L, Baum N *et al.* Safety and efficacy of mentor alpha-1 inflatable penile prosthesis for impotence treatment. *J Urol* 1997;157:833–9.

9. Levine LA, Guss SP. Gonaotropin-releasing hormone analogues in the treatment of sickle cell anemia-associated priapism. *J Urol* 1993;150:455–7.

10. Gupta S, Moreland RB, Munarriz R, Daley J, Goldstein I, Saenz de Tejada I. Possible role of Na-K-ATPase in the regulation of human corpus cavernosum smooth muscle contractility by nitric oxide. *Br J Pharmacol* 1995;116:2201–6.

11. Gupta S, Daley J, Pabby A, Hamaway K *et al.* A new mechanism for digoxin-associated impotence: in vitro and in vivo study. *J Urol* 1996;155:621(Abstract).

12. Belker AM, Thomas AJ, Fuchs EF *et al.* Results of 1,469 microsurgical vasectomy reversals by the vasovasotomy study group. *J Urol* 1991;145:505.

13. Brinsden PR, Wada I, Tan SL, Balen A, Jacobs HS. Diagnosis, prevention and management of ovarian hyperstimulation syndrome. *Brit J Ob Gyn* 1995;102:767–72.

14. Schlegel PN, Palermo GD, Goldstein M *et al.* Testicular sperm extraction with intracytoplasmic sperm injection for non-obstructive azoospermia. *Urology* 1997;49: 435–40.

15. Jarow JP, Sigman M, Buch JP, Oates RD. Delayed appearance of sperm after end-to-side vasoepididymostomy. *J Urol* 1995;153:1156–8.

16. Pavlovich CP, Schlegel PN. Fertility options after vasectomy: a cost-effectiveness analysis. *Fertil Steril* 1997;67:133–41.

17. Donovan JF, DiBaise AE, Kessler JA, Sandlow JI. Is vas reconstruction worth the effort? Comparison of repeat microscopic reconstruction of the vas following failed vasectomy reversal and advanced reproductive techniques. *Fertil Steril* 1997;Suppl S35;O-069.

18. Zonszein J. Diagnosis and management of endocrine disorders of erectile dysfunction. *Urol Clin N Am* 1995;22:789–802.

19. Morales A, Johnston B, Heaton JP, Lundie M. Testosterone supplementation for hypogonadal impotence: assessment of biochemical measures and therapeutic outcomes. *J Urol* 1997;157:849–54.

Urodynamics

DC Chaikin and JG Blaivas

The UroCenter of New York, and Cornell Medical Center, New York Hospital, New York, USA

Lower urinary tract symptoms in men

In 1997, urodynamics continued to be a major diagnostic tool in the diagnosis of lower urinary tract symptoms (LUTS; Table 1). Before the emergence of urodynamics, most clinicians used the words 'BPH', 'prostatism' and 'prostatic obstruction' interchangeably; however, it has been repeatedly shown that only half to two-thirds of patients actually have obstruction. The remainder have detrusor instability, impaired detrusor contractility, sensory urgency or polyuria. (The last two causes are rarely mentioned).

TABLE 1

Lower urinary tract symptoms

- Bladder outlet obstruction
- Impaired detrusor contractility
- Polyuria
- Nocturia
- Sensory urgency

Precise criteria for the urodynamic diagnosis of urethral obstruction was a focus of much investigation and there is a great deal of interest to find 'simple' urodynamic tests to predict treatment outcomes. Bruskewitz *et al.* evaluated symptoms score, uroflow, post-void residual urine and cystoscopy as predictors of outcome for transurethral resection of the prostate (TURP) and concluded that only the symptom score was a valid predictor.[1]

Of course, the relationship between detrusor pressure and uroflow remains the only valid means of diagnosing bladder outlet obstruction. A sustained detrusor contraction of adequate pressure associated with a low flow defines obstruction. In principle, all experts agree with this. They disagree, however, on:

- the exact pressure-flow cut-off point for urethral obstruction and impaired detrusor contractility
- exactly how to perform pressure-flow studies (i.e. the actual technique

used and the parameters measured)[2]

- perhaps most importantly, the relationship between urethral obstruction and LUTS and whether it is necessary to relieve obstruction to alleviate symptoms.

Computer models such as the linear passive urethral relation or the Abrams–Griffith nomogram certainly help the experienced urodynamacist in equivocal cases.[3] Nevertheless, at present, neither computer models nor 'simple tests' are able to substitute for the urodynamacist. In the series by Bruskewitz et al., only 71% of 245 patients symptomatically improved following TURP.[1] These numbers are consistent with previous reports on outcomes following TURP in patients who were not evaluated with urodynamics prior to surgery. A basic problem with this and most other studies on outcomes and urodynamic parameters is that the patients were not stratified with respect to severity. For example, men with severe obstruction, as evidenced by urodynamic criteria, might do much better than those with equivocal obstruction. We believe this to be true, though it remains to be proven. Furthermore, it should be recognized that many patients might seek treatment for symptoms that are caused by conditions unrelated to the lower urinary tract, e.g. polyuria, and this must be taken into account.

A number of investigations focused on the significance and bothersomeness of LUTS, and the impact pharmacological and surgical treatments have on these symptoms. Results indicate that neither the presence nor the severity of individual symptoms correlated with how bothersome they were.

- Peters et al. showed that "the symptoms that bother men the most are not the most common symptoms". Hesitancy and intermittency were the most common symptoms, but incontinence caused the most bother.[4]
- Jacobsen et al. showed that the incidence of urinary retention was low, but increased as LUTS increased.[5]
- Comiter et al. showed that LUTS could not reliably predict patients likely to progress to azotaemia.[6]
- Witjes et al. showed that men with LUTS can be successfully treated with alpha blockers. Patients who were obstructed according to urodynamic criteria, as well as those who were not obstructed, benefited from treatment.[7]

Highlights in **Urodynamics** 1997

WHAT'S IN ?

- Detrusor pressure/uroflow studies
- Computerized indices of urethral obstruction and impaired detrusor contractility
- Videourodynamics
- Leak point pressure
- Surgery
- Voiding questionnaires

WHAT'S OUT ?

- Urethral closure pressure profile
- Routine sphincter EMG

- Madersbacher *et al.* could not correlate International Prostate Symptom Score (IPSS) with the diagnosis of bladder outlet obstruction. Of patients with a maximum flow rate < 15 ml/second and IPSS > 7, 44% were unobstructed using the linear passive urethral resistance relation.[8]

These studies suggest that symptoms do not correlate with urodynamics diagnoses. In addition, they do not support the hypothesis that urethral obstruction causes symptoms and that relieving obstruction is a necessary correlate to relieving symptoms. What does this mean? Does it mean that urodynamics are not necessary or useful? We think just the opposite. The use of urodynamics in patients who have 'soft symptoms' should make it possible to characterize the aetiology of symptoms even more precisely. We believe that treatment aimed at the underlying pathophysiology is more likely to be effective than empirical treatment. But we may be wrong! Good clinical studies that stratify patients according to symptoms and urodynamic diagnoses and then treat them in a rational way need to be done. There is no reason to believe that a treatment aimed at 'unobstructing' a non-obstructed man will relieve nocturia due to excessive nocturnal production of urine!

Furthermore, you would think that by now, urologists would know whether or not it is necessary to treat obstruction in order to relieve symptoms. We don't. Remember, "if the only tool you have is a hammer, everything looks like a nail".

Incontinence

For most men and women with urinary incontinence, visual inspection of urinary loss from the urethra during provocation (e.g. cough or strain) is still the most obvious means of making the diagnosis when combined with good history-taking, diaries and pad tests. The recognition of the multifactorial nature of both post-prostatectomy incontinence and female incontinence is an important principle and urodynamics is an essential component in making the proper diagnosis.

Hammerer and Huland, in a prospective study of 82 patients undergoing radical retropubic and perineal prostatectomy, showed the multifactorial nature of incontinence.[9] All patients underwent urodynamics before and after radical prostatectomy. Pre-operatively, none had sphincteric incontinence and 17% had detrusor instability. Post-operatively, 41% had detrusor instability at 6–8 weeks and maximum urethral pressure fell from 90 to 65 cmH_2O. Functional length fell from 61 mm pre-operatively to 26 mm post-operatively. At 1 year, 9% of all patients had persistent incontinence, but no data were given to describe the aetiology.

In 1997, the diagnosis of intrinsic sphincter deficiency was most often made according to the leak point pressure (LPP) as well as clinical observation, but the technique of LPP remains to be standardized. Comiter *et al.* introduced retrograde measurement of the LPP. This technique uses X-rays to determine the pressure at which fluid infused into the distal urethra 'leaks' retrogradely into the bladder. They were able to perform measurements quickly and in a reproducible fashion. Results showed that the LPP was the same, whether standard methods were used or measurement was done retrogradely.[10] Cummings *et al.* showed that 54% of women evaluated for stress incontinence had a low LPP (< 65 cmH_2O), but had no traditional risk factors (previous incontinence surgery, radiation, etc.) for intrinsic sphincter deficiency. Consequently, it is important that these patients are identified so that the physician can recommend the most effective treatment, such as urethral bulking agent or a sling procedure.[11]

In addition, the finding that a low LPP does coexist with urethral hypermobility raises the question as to whether urethral hypermobility is a cause or accompaniment to stress injury incontinence.

Sanchez-Ortiz et al. showed that the LPP was an important predictor of success in men treated with periurethral collagen for post-prostatectomy incontinence.[12] Men with LPP > 60 cmH_2O were more likely to have a successful outcome than those whose LPP was lower. Patients with a good clinical outcome had a mean LPP of 64 cmH_2O, compared with 42 cmH_2O in the patients with a poor outcome. There was no difference between the groups with respect to severity of symptoms or number of pads used pre-operatively. The sensitivity of LPP as a treatment outcome predictor was 64% with a specificity of 85%; the overall positive predictive value of an LPP > 60 cmH_2O was 70% and the negative predictive value was 81%.

Concomitant pelvic relaxation in women can affect micturition sufficiently to alter voiding dynamics, which may cause LUTS or possibly mask incontinence. Coates et al. were able to show the multifactorial nature of female incontinence and the effect pelvic prolapse had on uroflowmetry.[13] Patients with pelvic prolapse had significantly lower flow rates compared with women with incontinence alone. It would be logical to assume that the prolapse was causing urethral obstruction in these patients, but this needs to be confirmed by pressure-flow studies. When performing urodynamics in patients with pelvic prolapse it is important to reduce the prolapse in order to assess micturition in this 'unobstructed' state, as well as to visualize any contributing incontinence which might affect outcome if surgery were to be performed.

Ambulatory urodynamics

Ambulatory monitoring did not receive much attention in 1997. Of course, the chance of detecting detrusor instability is greater with ambulatory monitoring than with conventional cystometry, if for no other reason than patients are monitored for a longer period of time.[14] Certainly, there must be improved standardization of those findings that are clinically meaningful.

Neurogenic bladder

The search continues to distinguish the neurogenic bladder from the non-neurogenic. Ronzoni et al. reported on the ice-water test.[15] This is an age-old test that is very little used in diagnosis of the neurogenic bladder today. The authors found an excellent sensitivity and specificity for neurologic lesions, though it is unclear whether anything is added to the information already obtained from urodynamic investigations.

Gray *et al.* showed that the characteristics of detrusor overactivity in the patient with neurologic damage are different from those in the neurologically intact patient.[16] This suggests differences between the pathophysiology and aetiology of the unstable bladder in the neurologically disabled patient and the intact patient, and certainly deserves further consideration.

References

1. Bruskewitz RC, Reda DJ, Wasson JH, Barrett L, Phelan M. Testing to predict outcome after transurethral resection of the prostate. *J Urol* 1997;157:1304–8.

2. Walker RMH, Di Pasquale B, Hubregtse M, St Clair Carter S. Pressure-flow studies in the diagnosis of bladder outlet obstruction: a study comparing suprapubic and transurethral techniques. *Br J Urol* 1997;79:693–7.

3. Trucchi A, Franco G, Manieri C, Valenti M, Carter SC, Tubaro A. Manual versus computer methods for diagnosing obstruction from pressure-flow tracings in patients with benign prostatic hyperplasia. *J Urol* 1997;157:871–5.

4. Peters SJ, Donovan JL, Kay HE *et al.* The International Continence Society "Benign Prostatic Hyperplasia" Study: the bothersomeness of urinary symptoms. *J Urol* 1997;157:885–9.

5. Jacobsen SJ, Jacobson DJ, Girman CJ *et al.* Natural history of prostatism: risk factors for acute urinary retention. *J Urol* 1997;158:481–7.

6. Comiter CV, Sullivan MP, Schacterle RS, Cohen LH, Yalla SV. Urodynamic risk factors for renal dysfunction in men with obstructive and nonobstructive voiding dysfunction. *J Urol* 1997;158: 181–5.

7. Witjes WPJ, Rosier PFWM, Caris CTM, Debruyne FMJ, De La Rosette JJMCH. Urodynamic and clinical effects of terazosin therapy in symptomatic patients with and without bladder outlet obstruction: a stratified analysis. *Urol* 1997;49:197–206.

8. Madersbacher S, Klinger HC, Djavan B *et al.* Is obstruction predictable by clinical evaluation in patients with lower urinary tract symptoms? *Br J Urol* 1997;80:72–7.

9. Hammerer P, Huland H. Urodynamic evaluation of changes in urinary control after radical retropubic prostatectomy. *J Urol* 1997;157:233–6.

10. Comiter CV, Sullivan MP, Yalla SV. Retrograde leak point pressure for evaluating postradical prostatectomy incontinence. *Urol* 1997;49:231–6.

11. Cummings JM, Boullier JA, Parra RO, Wozniak-Petrofsky J. Leak point pressures in women with urinary stress incontinence: correlation with patient history. *J Urol* 1997;157:818–20.

12. Sanchez-Ortiz RF, Broderick GA, Chaikin DC *et al*. Collagen injection therapy for post-radical retropubic prostatectomy incontinence: role of the valsalva leak point pressure. *J Urol* 1997; In press.

13. Coates KW, Harris RL, Cundiff GW, Bump RC. Uroflowmetry in women with urinary incontinence and pelvic organ prolapse. *Br J Urol* 1997;80:217–21.

14. Heslington K. Ambulatory bladder monitoring: is it an advance? *Br J Urol* 1997;80:49–53.

15. Ronzoni G, Menchinelli P, Manca A, De Giovanni L. The ice-water test in the diagnosis and treatment of the neurogenic bladder. *Br J Urol* 1997;79:698–701.

16. Gray R, Wagg A, Malone-Lee JG. Differences in detrusor contractile function in women with neuropathic and idiopathic detrusor instability. *Br J Urol* 1997;80:222–6.

Incontinence

PJR Shah

Institute of Urology and Nephrology, London, UK

Anatomy and physiology

Neural innervation. A neuroanatomical study of cadaveric female adult pelves has demonstrated an intrapelvic somatic pathway from S_{2-4} that supplies the levator ani and urethra.[1] These fibres lie beneath the endopelvic fascia, are distinct from the peripheral pudendal nerve, and lie in close proximity to the lateral and anterior vaginal wall. As a result, Borirakchanyavat et al. suggest that surgical techniques may need to be modified to preserve such innervation during radical pelvic surgery.

Pelvic floor. In a major review, Bernstein reported the results of a study of the pelvic floor muscles in women using perineal ultrasonography.[2] He admits that such an investigation is not easy to perform and that there was inter-observer variation in the results recorded. However, pelvic floor muscles were thicker in healthy women than in those with incontinence and the elderly, and Bernstein was able to demonstrate that a 6-month course of pelvic floor exercises led to an increase in the thickness of the pelvic floor muscles, both at rest and during contraction. Both previous gynaecological surgery and hysterectomy were more likely to be associated with urinary incontinence. Bernstein was also unable to demonstrate oestrogen receptors in the pelvic floor muscles, and it is suggested that a direct effect of oestrogen on the pelvic floor muscles is unlikely.

Psychosocial factors may influence the outcome of surgery for stress incontinence.[3] Women in whom surgery failed to cure incontinence have been shown to have a high degree of neuroticism, a low degree of extroversion, and anxiety. As a result, it is recommended that female candidates for surgery for stress incontinence should receive psychosocial support if optimal results are to be obtained.

Pregnancy is associated with a high incidence of stress incontinence (64%).[4]

Highlights in **Incontinence** *1997*

WHAT'S IN (STILL) ?

- Pelvic floor exercises
- Slings of various sorts
- Colposuspension
- Artificial urinary sphincters
- Injectables – collagen and Macroplastique

WHAT'S GAINING POPULARITY ?

- Bone anchors

WATCH THIS SPACE

- Intra-urethral inserts

WHAT SEEMS TO BE GOING OUT ?

- Needle suspensions except the 4-corner suspension

WHAT'S OUT ?

- Autologous fat
- Laparoscopic colposuspension

Furthermore, previous forceps delivery and multiparity are associated with a higher incidence of incontinence. Although pelvic floor function could easily be assessed during vaginal examination in pregnancy, this is not being done and, therefore, the opportunity to strengthen the pelvic floor muscles through exercise is being lost.

Irritable bowel syndrome and bladder instability have been shown to share certain symptomatic features, which may indicate a common underlying dysfunction.[5]

Investigation of incontinence

The classification of stress incontinence described by Blaivas[6] is still not used universally. Many patients undergo what are considered to be routine procedures for incontinence, such as colposuspension or needle suspension, when an alternative procedure is likely to produce a more effective result.

Valsalva leak point pressures are being used increasingly to provide information about intrinsic sphincter function,[7] and should become part of routine urodynamic testing prior to surgery for stress incontinence. Women with pelvic floor prolapse are more likely to have voiding dysfunction than those with urge incontinence, when assessed by flowmetry and volume of post-void residual urine.[8] However, routine urodynamic testing in women being considered for surgical treatment would enable each of the relevant features of bladder function to be recorded, which may have a bearing on selection of the procedure and the determination of outcome.

Conservative therapy for incontinence

Regular use of vaginal cones improves pelvic floor strength in healthy women and those with stress and urge incontinence.[9] Even women with no discernible pelvic floor contraction improve with the regular use of vaginal cones. Pelvic floor exercises may also help men with post-micturition dribbling, which can be a very distressing symptom. Paterson *et al.* showed that pelvic floor exercises were more effective than urethral milking in these men, demonstrating that improving the strength of the bulbo-perineal muscles has a role to play in the treatment of this common benign condition.[10]

The symptoms of frequency and urgency after prostatectomy may be significantly reduced by treatment with oxybutynin during the first week after surgery.[11]

Injectable agents for stress incontinence

A number of injectable agents are available for the treatment of stress incontinence and, each year, a number of publications report the longer-term results of individual experiences. It does appear, however, that injectable agents will have a role for some time, because patients still find the concept of a pain-free, day-case procedure with a reasonable chance of success attractive.

Experimental procedures with potential. Yoo *et al.* inserted an inflatable self-sealing membrane below the urethral mucosa in female dogs.[12] They found the membrane to be encapsulated and static after a period of up to 18 months. They therefore suggest that such a device may provide an alternative to the injectable materials currently available.

Autologous fat injected into the urethra has been reported to have little success in the long term. Although Palma *et al.* have produced results which suggest a 64% cure rate in 11 patients after 1 year of follow-up,[13] it is possible that, in time, they will experience the same failure rate as other investigators. Therefore, further long-term reports of the use of autologous fat should be awaited before it is adopted as an alternative to commercially available agents.

Collagen is still popular and continues to be the subject of a significant number of publications. Smith *et al.* reported that, using an average of 2.1 procedures and 11.9 ml collagen, 67% of 84 patients achieved continence at a median follow-up of 14 months.[14] The transurethral route of injection has produced a higher success rate than the periurethral route, as placement of the injectable agent is more accurate and the re-treatment rate is lower.[15] In patients with incontinence treated with collagen, 61% were patients reported as being 'satisfied' at 4-year follow-up.[16]

Macroplastique. A single treatment with Macroplastique provides successful resolution of stress incontinence in 90% of patients at 1 month, falling to 75% at 3 months and 48% after 2 years.[17] The low success rate at 2 years was influenced by the inclusion of patients with significant bladder base descent (type II). Treatment with Macroplastique does not, however, appear to be successful in patients with type II incontinence. Furthermore, in patients with significant prolapse, repositioning or supporting procedures are more appropriate and injectable agents should be avoided.

Injectable agents in men. Transurethral collagen for the treatment of post-prostatectomy incontinence did not produce encouraging results according to Griebling et al.[18] The situation has, however, been clarified by Chaikin et al., who used Valsalva leak point pressure (LPP) measurements to assess the effects of collagen injections in post-prostatectomy incontinence.[19] Where the LPP was greater than 60 cmH$_2$O, the likelihood of success was much greater, but injection volumes of up to 28 ml with a mean of 2.6 injections/patient were required.

Surgical procedures

One would imagine that the surgery for stress incontinence would, by now, have been sufficiently defined and established so that little new could be devised. However, a number of new or modified techniques have been presented or published in 1997, with an increasing emphasis on the various sling procedures.

Burch colposuspension is still considered the treatment of choice by some surgeons.[20] Following this procedure, approximately 80% of patients may be expected to be dry or markedly improved after 10 years. Enterocele (19%) and urgency (37%) are the main long-term problems.

Laparoscopic procedures have been criticized for the duration of the procedure and results that do not match those of colposuspension, which has been well proven. Nevertheless, satisfactory results with reduced morbidity have been reported using laparoscopic procedures, particularly those using endoscopic staples.[21] However, when the results of laparoscopy are followed for more than a year, the success rate appears to fall considerably; Breda et al. found that the success rate fell to 68.6% after nearly 3 years.[22] Thus, although laparoscopy appears to be associated with a lower morbidity than open colposuspension, it has once again been confirmed as less effective in the longer term.

Pubovaginal slings have provided much interest this year. The choice of sling material varies from centre to centre – fascia lata,[23] rectus fascia,[24,25] and vaginal wall[26,27] have all been reported (Table 1).

A comparison of a fascia lata sling with collagen in the treatment of stress incontinence by Berman and Kreder suggested that the sling may be a more cost-effective, long-term solution.[28] Although the cost of the sling procedure

TABLE 1

Studies of pubovaginal slings – a review

Type of sling	Study	Number of patients	Success rate (%)
Fascia lata	Govier et al.[23]	32	87
Rectus fascia	Carr et al.[24]	19	100
Rectus fascia	Fulford et al.[25]	85	78
Vaginal wall	Litwiller et al.[26]	42	74
Vaginal wall	Rovner et al.[27]	413	93

was 2.1 times greater, its success rate at 21 months was 71.4% compared with 26.7% for collagen. Quality of life after sling surgery has been considered by Hassounna and Ghoneim;[29] 79% of patients reported an improvement in social activities and 40.5% in sexual activity.

Blaivas et al. consider the pubovaginal sling to be an effective treatment for "all types of incontinence".[30] However, those with urethral scarring and persistent detrusor instability were likely to have the worst outcome. This group found a success rate of 86% after long-term follow-up for 5 years.

Bone anchors provide stable fixation of sutures when open or endoscopic procedures for stress incontinence are used,[31] and appear to produce short-term results similar, in terms of efficacy, to those achieved with the Stamey procedure.

The artificial urinary sphincter

Long-term concerns about the efficacy and durability of the AUS800 were raised in 1996. There is no doubt that patients who have had artificial sphincters for over 15 years will almost certainly have had the device revised, replaced or removed for various complications. This should signify concern about the insertion of these devices in younger people. Fulford et al. in Cardiff reported their long-term experience with the AUS800.[32] Of 61 patients, 49 patients had required at least one revision and only 8 patients had original functioning sphincters. Nevertheless, 61% of patients were continent after 10 years with an implanted AMS800.

Successful cure of incontinence has been achieved with the AMS800 in

89% of women with intractable stress incontinence.[33] One of the major advantages of the artificial sphincter in this group of patients was avoiding the need for clean-intermittent self-catheterization.

Guidelines for the surgical management of stress incontinence

The Female Stress Urinary Incontinence Clinical Guidelines Panel of the American Urological Association found that surgery offered long-term cure in a significant proportion of patients. Open colposuspension and slings were found to be more effective than needle suspensions, though they had a slightly higher morbidity.[34]

References

1. Borirakchanyavat S, Aboseif SR, Carroll PR, Tanagho EA, Lue TF. Continence mechanism of the isolated female urethra: an anatomical study of the intrapelvic somatic nerves. *J Urol* 1997;158:822–6.

2. Bernstein IT. The pelvic floor muscles: muscle thickness in healthy and urinary-incontinent women measured by perineal ultrasonography with reference to the effect of pelvic floor training. Estrogen receptor studies. *Neurourol Urodyn* 1997;16:237–75.

3. Berglund AL, Eisemann M, Lalos A, Lalos O. Predictive factors of the outcome of primary surgical treatment of stress incontinence in women. *Scand J Urol Nephrol* 1997;31(1):49–55.

4. Chiarelli P, Campbell E. Incontinence during pregnancy. Prevalence and opportunities for continence promotion. *Aust NZ J Obstet Gynaecol* 1997;37:66–73.

5. Cukier JM, Cortina-Borja M, Brading AF. A case-control study to examine any association between idiopathic detrusor instability and gastrointestinal tract disorder, and between irritable bowel syndrome and urinary tract disorder. *Br J Urol* 1997;79:865–78.

6. Blaivas JG, Olsson CA. Stress incontinence: classification and surgical approach. *J Urol* 1988;139:727–31.

7. Cummings JM, Boullier JA, Parra RO, Wozniak-Petrofsky J. Leak point pressures in women with urinary stress incontinence: correlation with patient history. *J Urol* 1997;157:818–20.

8. Coates KW, Harris RL, Cundiff GW, Bump RC. Uroflowmetry in women with urinary incontinence and pelvic organ prolapse. *Br J Urol* 1997;80:217–21.

9. Fischer W, Linde A. Pelvic floor findings in urinary incontinence – results of conditioning using vaginal cones. *Acta Obstet Gynecol Scand* 1997;76(5):455–60.

10. Paterson J, Pinnock CB, Marshall VR. Pelvic floor exercises as a treatment for post-micturition dribble. *Br J Urol* 1997;79(6):892–7.

11. Iselin CE, Schmidlin F, Borst F, Rohner S, Graber P. Oxybutynin in the treatment of early detrusor instability after transurethral resection of the prostate. *Br J Urol* 1997;79:915–19.

12. Yoo JJ, Magliochetti M, Atala A. Detachable self-sealing membrane system for the endoscopic treatment of incontinence. *J Urol* 1997;158:1045–8.

13. Palma PC, Riccetto CL, Herrmann V, Netto NR Jr. Repeated lipoinjections for stress urinary incontinence. *J Endourol* 1997;1:67–70.

14. Smith DN, Appell RA, Winters JC, Rackley RR. Collagen injection therapy for female intrinsic sphincteric deficiency. *J Urol* 1997;157:1275–8.

15. Litwiller SE, Nelson RS, Stone AR. Comparison of transurethral and periurethral collagen – a comparison of outcome and patient satisfaction. *J Urol* 1997;157:458(Abstract).

16. Corcos J, Fournier C. 4-year follow-up of collagen injection for urinary stress incontinence. *J Urol* 1997;157:458 (Abstract).

17. Sheriff MKM, Foley S, Mcfarlane J, Nauth-Misir R, Shah PJR. Endoscopic correction of intractable stress incontinence with silicone micro-implants. *Eur Urol* 1997;32:284–8.

18. Griebling TL, Kreder KJ Jr, Williams RD. Transurethral collagen injection for treatment of postprostatectomy urinary incontinence in men. *Urology* 1997;49 (6):907–12.

19. Chaikin DC, Broderick GA, Blander DS, Sanchez-Ortiz R, Malkowitz B, Wein AJ. Collagen therapy for post-prostatectomy incontinence: the role of the Valsalva leak point pressure. *J Urol* 1997;157:185(Abstract).

20. Laine M, Kiilholma P, Makinen J. Long-term results of colposuspension. *J Urol* 1997;157:265(Abstract).

21. Lyons TL, Winer WK. Clinical outcomes with laparoscopic approaches and open Burch procedures for urinary stress incontinence. *J Am Assoc Gynecol Laparosc* 1995;2(2):193–8.

22. Breda G, Silvestre P, Tamai A, Gherardi L, Xausa D, Guinta A. Laparoscopic surgery of stress urinary incontinence in women. *Chir Ital* 1996;48:35–40.

23. Govier FE, Gibbons RP, Correa RJ, Weissman RM, Pritchett TR, Hefty TR. Pubovaginal slings using fascia lata for the treatment of intrinsic sphincter deficiency. *J Urol* 1997;157:117–21.

24. Carr LK, Walsh PJ, Abraham VE, Webster GD. Favorable outcome of pubovaginal slings for geriatric women with stress incontinence. *J Urol* 1997;157:125–8.

25. Fulford S, Flynn R, Stephenson TP. A subjective and urodynamic assessment of the rectus fascial sling with particular reference to the urge syndrome. *Br J Urol* 1997;79:214.

26. Litwiller SE, Nelson RS, Fone PD, Kim KB, Stone AR. Vaginal wall sling: long-term outcome analysis of factors contributing to patient satisfaction and surgical success. *J Urol* 1997;157: 1279–82.

27. Rovner ES, Ginsberg DA, Raz S. Vaginal wall sling for anatomical incontinence and intrinsic sphincter dysfunction: an update on efficacy and long-term outcome. *J Urol* 1997;157: 266.

28. Berman CJ, Kreder KJ. Comparative cost analysis of collagen injection and fascia lata sling cystourethropexy for the treatment of type III incontinence in women. *J Urol* 1997;157:122–4.

29. Hassouna M, Ghoneim GM. Short- and long-term outcome and patient satisfaction following modified pubo-vaginal sling (MPVS) for stress urinary incontinence. *J Urol* 1997;157:187 (Abstract).

30. Blaivas JG, Romanzi L. Pubo-vaginal sling (PVS) for all types of stress incontinence (SUI): long-term follow-up of 251 patients.

31. Morley R, Cumming J, Birch B. Staple colpofixation: a new minimally invasive treatment for stress incontinence. *J Urol* 1997;157:457 (Abstract).

32. Fulford SCV, Sutton C, Bales G, Hickling M, Stephenson TP. The fate of the 'modern' artificial urinary sphincter with a follow-up of more than 10 years. *Br J Urol* 1997;79:713–6.

33. Schreiter F, Heitz M. The artificial urinary sphincter AMS800 in the female: indication and results in 161 patients. *J Urol* 1997;157:459(Abstract).

34. Leach GE, Dmochowski RR, Appell RA *et al.* Female stress urinary incontinence clinical guidelines panel summary report on surgical management of female stress urinary incontinence. *J Urol* 1997;158:875–80.

Paediatric urology

LS Baskin

UCSF Children's Medical Center, University of California, San Francisco, USA

Hypospadias – anatomy

In a recent study, normal human fetal penile specimens and a human fetal hypospadiac specimen were serially sectioned and stained by immunohistochemical techniques to locate nerves and vascular structures.[1] The nerves in both the normal and hypospadiac specimens of all age ranges were most commonly found at the classic positions of 11 o'clock and 1 o'clock, but also extended completely around the tunica to the junction of the urethral spongiosum and corpora cavernosa (Figure 1); no nerves were noted at the 12 o'clock position, which has not been reported previously in the postnatal penis. The neuro-anatomy of the hypospadiac penis was similar to the normal fetal penis, except for the abnormal hypospadiac glandular area and the underside of the urethral plate, which was characterized by numerous large blood-filled sinuses. These vascular sinuses extended from just underneath the skin to the corporal bodies, which

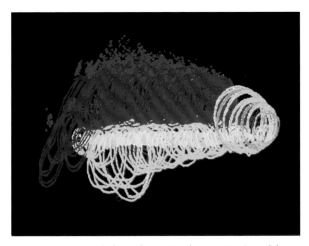

Figure 1 A computer-generated, three-dimensional reconstruction of the normal human fetal penis at 25 weeks' gestation. Nerves = red; tunica = blue; urethral lumen = yellow; urethral spongiosum and prepuce = green.

appeared normal. Proximal to the hypospadiac meatus, the vascular sinuses resolved into a normal urethral spongiosum.

The location of the nerves has implications for the design of penile strengthening procedures and feminizing genitoplasty reconstruction. The extensive vascular sinuses of the hypospadiac penis under the exact area of the tubularized incised plate urethroplasty shed some light on why this procedure may produce excessive bleeding. Extensive vascular channels with endothelial cell linings and nutrient supply may explain the reported success of incising the urethral plate with primary tubularization. The fact that no nerves are present in the 12 o'clock position also allows for an anatomical approach to straightening penile curvature by placing parallel plication sutures in the exact midline where they will not disturb any of the neurovascular anatomy (Figure 2).

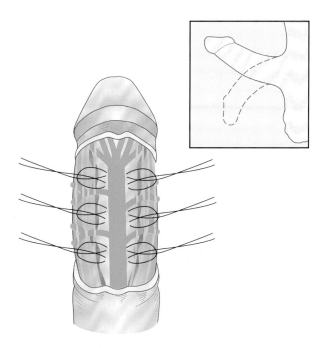

Figure 2 Multiple parallel suture plication technique at the 12.00 o'clock position for the correction of ventral curvature in patients with hypospadias and congenital penile curvature.

Highlights in **Paediatric urology** 1997

NEW CONCEPTS

- Penile neurovascular anatomy: implications for penile straightening
- Testicular microlithiasis
- Spiral CT scan for the evaluation of urinary tract reconstruction
- The prepuce is not the only culprit in UTIs

CLASSIC CONCEPTS

- Prophylaxis for vesico-ureteral reflux
- Torsion of the undescended testis: relation to hCG administration
- Decreased fertility in formerly unilateral cryptorchid males
- Careful testicular exam under anaesthesia prior to laparoscopy
- Variations of the onlay island flap for hypospadias

Testicular microlithiasis

Testicular microlithiasis is usually diagnosed by the presence of diffuse, intraparenchymal, hyperechoic foci, 1–3 mm in diameter, on testicular ultrasound. Although it is usually a rare condition in children, the widespread use of testicular ultrasound has resulted in an increased number of cases being discovered incidentally. In adults, both benign and malignant conditions have been associated with testicular microlithiasis; an association with germ cell tumours is seen in up to 40% of cases. The natural history of testicular microlithiasis found incidentally in children is not well defined.

In a retrospective study that analysed the records of patients with incidentally discovered testicular microlithiasis from six centres, 20 of the 25 patients were found to have bilateral disease.[2] The scrotal conditions that prompted the testicular ultrasound included: orchalgia or acute pain (n = 6); hydrocele (n = 5); epididymitis/orchitis (n = 5); testicular mass or size discrepancy (n = 4); varicocele (n = 3); and scrotal trauma (n = 2); average age of presentation was 12.3 years (range 6 months to 21 years).

Measurements of tumour markers, α-fetoprotein and β-human chorionic gonadotrophin (hCG) were available for 15 patients and all were normal. Testicular biopsy was performed in 9 patients and showed dystrophic calcifications without evidence of malignancy or abnormal seminiferous tubules. Follow-up, which ranged from 1 month to 7 years, comprised annual testicular ultrasound and clinical examination and revealed no evidence of testicular tumours.

The authors concluded that testicular microlithiasis in children shows no trend towards malignant degeneration. However, they feel that the length of follow-up may be insufficient to detect tumour development and advocate surveillance, with annual testicular ultrasound, physical examination and, perhaps, measurement of testicular tumour markers. They also propose that a register should be established to follow patients with testicular microlithiasis in order to define its significance in childhood.

Evaluation following continent reconstruction

Patients with spina bifida require long-term urological surveillance, because of the risk of hydronephrosis, renal and reservoir calculi, and renal infection and scarring following urinary tract construction. This can be challenging because of associated spinal anomalies and body habitus.

Elder *et al.* investigated the use of non-contrast spiral CT scanning of the abdomen and pelvis with the aim of providing more accurate and faster imaging of the entire urinary tract than routine ultrasound.[3] A total of 13 patients, with neuropathic bladders and continent urinary tract reconstruction using intestine, underwent spiral CT scanning without contrast as part of a routine follow-up evaluation; 11 patients had an ultrasound examination for comparison. The spiral CT scan was performed in 10 minutes or less, which is shorter than the time required for ultrasonography. Delineation of the urinary tract and abdominal wall was superior with spiral CT in all patients, for example:

- only 19 of the 21 kidneys were identified by ultrasonography
- renal calculi were identified in two patients on CT, but were not seen on ultrasound
- in one patient, a bladder calculus that was identified on ultrasound turned out to be a uterine fibroid when analysed by spiral CT

- three patients had abdominal hernias that were not detected on physical examination.

Non-contrast CT scanning is, therefore, a fast, non-invasive and reliable method of visualizing the urinary tract and abdominal wall in patients with neurogenic abnormalities. Although this technique is unlikely to replace ultrasound in most patients, it is well suited to the evaluation of patients with complicated urinary tract reconstruction.

Circumcision and UTI

It is generally believed that the presence of a foreskin is a major determinant of urinary tract infection (UTI) in new-born boys. At St Louis University, USA, a group lead by Steinhardt prospectively examined the incidence of genitourinary anomalies in circumcised and uncircumcised boys who presented with their first UTI before 6 months of age.[4] Diagnosis of pyelonephritis was established on clinical grounds and required systemic complaints, such as fever, lethargy, leucocytosis and vomiting, to be present. All infants were evaluated by renal ultrasound and voiding cysto-urethrogram. Complete information was obtained on a total of 108 boys, of whom 52 were circumcised and 56 were uncircumcised. The distribution in each group with respect to race was identical: 79% of patients were Caucasian; 17% Afro-American; and 5% of Asian and Hispanic origin combined.

Imaging revealed normal anatomy in 26 of the 108 boys of whom 46% were circumcised and 54% uncircumcised. Abnormal anatomy was demonstrated in 77% of the circumcised boys and 75% of uncircumcised boys. There was no statistically significant difference between the two groups. Of the anatomical abnormalities, 70% were reflux, 21% obstruction, 4% Prune Belly syndrome, 3% valves and 2% bladder diverticulum. It was concluded that, regardless of circumcision status, infants who present with UTI during the first 6 months of life are likely to have an underlying genitourinary abnormality. In those infants without anatomical abnormalities, UTIs were found in as many circumcised infants as uncircumcised infants. Thus, all male infants presenting with UTI before 6 months of age should be investigated accordingly, irrespective of circumcision status or race.

Prophylaxis against UTI

The goal of treating patients with vesico-ureteral reflux is to prevent UTI until the reflux resolves spontaneously. Although Jean Smellie, in her classic studies, showed that low-dose, daily antibiotic prophylaxis could prevent UTI, this supposition has recently been questioned. In a study to establish whether close surveillance without the use of antibiotics could eliminate the need for long-term, daily antibiotic therapy,[5] children with newly diagnosed vesico-ureteral reflux were randomized into one of three groups:

- surveillance alone with no antibiotic prophylaxis, but daily testing of the urine for nitrites
- intermittent antibiotic prophylaxis with daily urine nitrite testing
- continuous antibiotic prophylaxis without tests, which is the current care standard.

All children underwent periodic DSMA scans to detect renal scars. Breakthrough UTIs were treated after obtaining a urine culture and the results of sensitivity testing. The demography of the three groups of patients was similar. The incidence of documented UTIs in the surveillance group was greater than that in either the continuous prophylaxis or the intermittent prophylaxis groups. One patient in the surveillance group had new renal parenchymal involvement (new scar) documented by DSMA scan.

This study confirms that the management of children with vesico-ureteral reflux with continuous prophylactic antibiotics or intermittent antibiotics is effective, and prevents UTI and renal injury. In contrast, the patients managed by dipstick surveillance had a higher incidence of UTIs and were also at risk of renal parenchymal injury. The financial costs of urinary dipstick surveillance was $US15/month compared with $US5/month for antibiotic prophylaxis. Surveillance of patients with vesico-ureteral reflux does not, therefore, seem to be cost-effective nor efficacious in preventing UTIs or preserving renal function.

Torsion of the undescended testis

The incidence of undescended testis at birth is approximately 3%, decreasing to 0.8% at 1 year of age. After 1 year, the incidence remains at 0.8%, implying that if a testicle is going to descend naturally, it will have done so by the first birthday. Anecdotal reports have suggested that patients who have cryptorchid testes are at higher risk of torsion and the Atlanta group in the USA has reviewed six cases of torsion of an undescended testis in terms of presentation, diagnosis and management.[6]

All the boys had a palpable unilateral or bilateral undescended testis, which was not considered to represent neonatal torsion or vanishing testes. They ranged in age from 5 months to 19 years (mean 4.2 years). Symptoms were acute in onset in all six boys and primarily consisted of irritability, vomiting and associated tender groin masses. Time of presentation ranged from 1 hour to 1 week; interestingly, two of the patients received hCG or testosterone by intramuscular injection in the 4–6 hours preceding the onset of symptoms. All six patients underwent surgical exploration, but only one of the six testes was successfully salvaged and the remaining five were removed.

It was concluded that patients with cryptorchidism are at risk of torsion while awaiting spontaneous descent. Presenting symptoms are often nonspecific and salvage of the testes is rare. It is therefore essential to warn patients and/or their parents of the risk of torsion, especially those being treated with intramuscular testosterone or hCG.

Fertility in unilateral cryptorchidism

Whether men with a history of unilateral cryptorchidism treated by orchidopexy have a higher incidence of infertility than men with normally descended testes is controversial. Lee *et al.* at the University of Pittsburgh, USA, are carrying out an ongoing prospective male fertility study in men with formerly cryptorchid testes and a group of age-matched controls.[7] Investigations include blood samples before and after stimulation with gonadotrophin-releasing hormone, measurement of luteinizing hormone, follicle-stimulating hormone (FSH) and testosterone, and analysis of sperm density, motility and morphology. Data from both the formerly unilateral cryptorchid group and the control group, and the men known to be fertile and infertile were compared.

Plasma FSH levels were higher and sperm counts lower among the formerly cryptorchid men than in the controls, suggesting compromised spermatogenesis. Among the patients with cryptorchidism, elevated FSH levels and low sperm counts were also suggestive of decreased fertility potential. This study further supports the decreased fertility potential in formerly unilateral cryptorchid men.

61

Diagnostic laparoscopy

The role of laparoscopy in paediatric urology remains undefined. Many advocate laparoscopy for the treatment of the non-palpable testis and in the investigation of patients with intersex abnormalities. Others feel that laparoscopy is time-consuming, expensive and of limited benefit in the paediatric age group.

The group at Boston Children's Hospital, USA, analysed their experience in patients with a non-palpable testis.[8] One of the main criticisms of laparoscopy is the frequent finding of an inguinal testis, which occurs in approximately 50% of these patients. The Boston group investigated the effect of a careful examination under anaesthesia on the number of unnecessary diagnostic laparoscopic procedures. Between 1992 and 1996, the authors retrospectively reviewed 259 non-palpable testes in 217 patients. Of these, 46 testes (18%) were found in 40 patients during examination under anaesthesia. The remaining 215 cases were considered appropriate for laparoscopic evaluation. Of the patients evaluated laparoscopically, only 14% had testes that could be considered missed on examination. In other words, they were visible distal to the ring, while 38% had intra-abdominal testes, 10% had vanishing testes, 11% had peeping testes, 37% had inguinal testes and 3% had scrotal knobbins. In the patients that underwent laparoscopy, 46% of the testes were found during the inguinal dissection.

Thus, in 46% of patients, it could be argued that laparoscopy provided no additional benefit over simple inguinal exploration, while exploration was avoided or limited as a result of laparoscopic findings in 14%. As examination under anaesthesia identified testes in 18% of the total group, which significantly reduced the number of uninformative laparoscopic procedures carried out, this step should not be omitted in patients who are scheduled for laparoscopic evaluation for non-palpable testes.

Split prepuce *in situ* on the hypospadias repair

Rushton and Belman from Children's Medical Center, Washington DC, USA, reported their experience of 100 consecutive patients with penile shaft hypospadias and chordee, who underwent a variation of the onlay island flap hypospadias repair.[9] Their technique involves splitting the inner and outer prepuce in the midline after measuring the length of tissue needed to form the urethra. The flap is swung ventrally and the under-surface of the

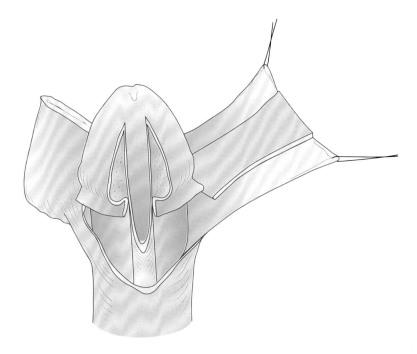

Figure 3 Split prepuce *in situ* technique for the onlay island flap repair in hypospadias.

prepuce is isolated as an island of de-epithelialized outer foreskin (Figure 3). After tailoring the remaining inner preputial island, it is sutured to the intact urethral plate to form the ventral aspect of the new urethra. Its pedicle consists of all the subcutaneous tissue from the half of the prepuce rather than only the inner layer as for the usual transverse island flap. The redundant subcutaneous tissue is then used to cover the neo-urethra.

Excellent cosmetic and functional results were obtained using this technique; only 3% of patients had a urethral fistula and no patients had meatal stenosis. Furthermore, the split prepuce *in situ* technique is simpler to perform than the traditional onlay, optimizes the blood supply and provides well-vascularized coverage of the neo-urethra.

References

1. Baskin LS, Erol A, Wu Li Y. Neuro and vascular anatomy of hypospadias: Why the Snodgrass bleeds and works. *Paediatrics* 1997;100(3):548.

2. Furness PD, Husman DA, Brock JW, Steinhardt GF, Bukowski TP, Freedman AL, Cheng EY. A multi-institutional study of testicular microlithiasis in children: a benign or premalignant condition? *Paediatrics* 1997;100(3):573.

3. Elder JS, Myers M, Sivit C. Spiral CT scan without contrast for evaluation of the urinary tract following continent reconstruction: preliminary report. *Paediatrics* 1997;100(3):567.

4. Mueller ER, Steinhardt G, Naseer S. The incidence of genitourinary abnormalities in circumcised and uncircumcised boys presenting with an initial urinary tract infection by 6 months of age. *Paediatrics* 1997;100(3):580.

5. Reddy PP, Evans MT, Hughes PA *et al.* Antimicrobial prophylaxis in children with vesico-ureteral reflux: a randomized prospective study of continuous therapy versus intermittent therapy versus surveillance. *Paediatrics* 1997;100 (3):555.

6. Riden DJ, Kalish J, Broecker BH, Massad CA, Woodard JR. Torsion of the undescended testis: a report of six cases. *Paediatrics* 1997;100(3):575.

7. Lee PA, Coughlin MT, Bellinger MF, O'Leary LA, Kalista C, LaPorte RE. Correlations between hormone levels, sperm parameters and paternity among formerly unilateral cryptorchid men. *Paediatrics* 1997;100(3):574.

8. Cisek LJ, Peters CA, Atala A, Bauer SB, Diamond DA, Retik AB. Improved outcomes in diagnostic laparoscopy of the nonpalpable testis. *Paediatrics* 1997;100(3):572.

9. Rushton HG, Belman B, Morgan TO. The split prepuce *in-situ* onlay hypospadias repair: the first 100 cases. *Paediatrics* 1997;100(3):72.

Neurourology

Ph EV Van Kerrebroeck

Department of Urology, University Hospital Maastricht, The Netherlands

In the past year, neurourological topics have been covered in numerous publications and at international meetings worldwide, reflecting an increasing interest in this area among urologists.

Diagnosis

Neurophysiological testing. The extent by which the descending sympathetic spinal tract was spared was studied and correlated with bladder neck function in spinal-cord-injured patients.[1] Sympathetic skin responses were recorded and found to be abnormal in all patients with a lesion above T6 and bladder neck dyssynergia associated with autonomic hyperreflexia. Thus, the integrity of the descending sympathetic spinal tract appears necessary for a synergistic function of the vesicourethral complex. Furthermore, sympathetic skin responses could be useful in the diagnosis of bladder neck dyssynergia in patients with a lesion above Th6.

Urodynamics. The 'old' ice-water test was revived in the urological literature. Two studies investigated the usefulness of this test in the diagnosis and treatment of neurogenic bladder dysfunction.[2,3] The first study included 130 patients with detrusor hyperreflexia and detrusor instability. The overall sensitivity in patients with detrusor hyperreflexia was 65% and the specificity was 85%, but only 46% of patients with suprapontine causes of detrusor hyperreflexia had a positive test.[2] Thus, the test was insufficiently sensitive to discriminate between detrusor hyperreflexia and detrusor instability. The second study found the test to be positive in 95% of patients with a complete medullary lesion and used it as a basis for further bladder rehabilitation.[3]

Another study compared the urodynamic indices of isometric and isotonic detrusor contractile function in patients with idiopathic detrusor instability and in patients with multiple sclerosis and detrusor hyperreflexia.[4] Storage, isometric detrusor contractile and voiding outflow functions were found to differ in the two conditions. Thus, it was concluded that these different types of detrusor instability may not share the same pathophysiological pathway.

Attention has also been paid to the effects of intervention on the behaviour of the bladder. A retrospective study obtained urodynamic data from 39 patients with a tethered spinal cord that was surgically released.[5] Two groups were distinguished; one with occult spinal dysraphism and another with secondary tethering after previous intervention. In the first group, hyperreflexia was the common finding and was resolved in 62.5% of patients after untethering. In the second group, impaired compliance was the most important finding and improved in only 30% of patients. It was concluded that early surgical intervention may improve urological symptoms and urodynamic patterns in patients with spinal dysraphism, but not in patients with secondary spinal cord tethering.

The effects of neuromodulation have been evaluated in a urodynamic study.[6] Of 27 patients with voiding dysfunction, 17 responded well to neuromodulation of the sacral nerves. All had a hypocontractile detrusor in combination with sphincter hypertonicity. In those not reacting, the contractility at diagnosis was significantly lower. In patients with preserved detrusor contractility, neuromodulation is a possible therapeutic option.

Therapy

Conservative. Two studies of the effects of chronic catheterization in patients with spinal cord injury were published. A long-term follow-up of a group of 84 female tetraplegics was presented.[7] Patients with complete lesions were difficult to manage – 85% were treated with indwelling catheters. However, patients with good functional recovery had better outcomes – most voided with controlled triggering or intermittent catheterization. In a group of 142 male patients with spinal cord injury, the long-term urological complications were monitored.[8] Urological complications occurred significantly more often in the catheterized group than in the non-catheterized group. There was also more renal damage in the catheterized group. The general conclusion is that elimination of indwelling urinary catheters will reduce the incidence of urinary tract complications and lead to better preservation of renal function.

For patients with bladder-emptying problems, a commercially available body massager appears to improve voiding in about 70% of patients with

Highlights in **Neurourology** 1997

WHAT'S IN ?

- Neuromodulation for voiding dysfunction
- Sacral anterior root stimulation in spinal cord injury

WHAT'S NEW ?

- Queen Square bladder stimulator

WHAT'S OUT ?

- Detrusor myotomy

OLD FAVOURITES

- Intravesical capsaicin

neurological diseases; it also reduced the post-voiding residual urine.[9] There were no complications and patients complied well.

Previous publications have dealt with the beneficial effects of capsaicin instillations to control neurogenic bladder overactivity. In a group of 14 patients, the urodynamic and clinical effects were studied.[10] Mean time to first desire to void and maximal cystometric capacity increased significantly. The effects lasted for 6–12 months and were renewed following repeat instillation.

Surgical. With a conservative approach, a group of patients with neurogenic disorders will present with persisting bladder problems. Many articles have focused on the effects of sacral rhizotomies, eventually in combination with sacral anterior root stimulation. From a single centre, long-term follow-up data with sacral anterior root stimulation have been presented.[11] Patients' quality of life appeared to increase markedly, but some experienced significant complications. A smaller study with the same type of stimulation had excellent results in terms of restoration of continence and disappearance of reflux.[12]

A study of 52 patients with spinal cord injury treated with sacral rhizotomies and electrical bladder stimulation analysed clinical and urodynamic parameters together with cost-effectiveness and quality of life.[13,14] Complete continence was achieved in 73% of patients during the day and in 86% at night. The incidence of urinary tract infections was reduced due to better bladder emptying. Although the initial costs with this treatment were high, they were recouped in 8 years. Patient satisfaction with bladder emptying increased and the problems of micturition and incontinence decreased significantly.

Current research aims at more selective stimulation of autonomic rootlets. Animal experiments have shown the feasibility of this technique, which spares somatic rootlets.[15] In recent years, evidence has shown that detrusor myotomy could be beneficial to patients with therapy-resistant detrusor overactivity. A recent article, however, reported disappointing results with this technique and cast doubt on the value of myotomy as a procedure for motor urge incontinence.[16]

Intermittent catheterization is an alternative treatment for patients with spinal cord injury. More commonly, an extra channel is made to facilitate catheterization; this can even be successful in patients with poor hand function. The 'Mitrofanoff umbilical appendicovesicostomy' is another treatment option that was studied in a group of seven patients with quadriplegia.[17] Following surgery, all patients were continent and able to self-catheterize, but two patients needed revision surgery.

References

1. Schurch B, Curt A, Rossier AB. The value of sympathetic skin response recordings in the assessment of the vesicourethral autonomic nervous dysfunction in spinal cord injured patients. *J Urol* 1997;157:2230–3.

2. Petersen T, Chandiramani V, Fowler CJ. The ice-water test in detrusor hyper-reflexia and bladder instability. *Br J Urol* 1997;79:163–7.

3. Ronzoni G, Menchinelli P, Manca A, De Giovanni L. The ice-water test in the diagnosis of the neurogenic bladder. *Br J Urol* 1997;79:698–701.

4. Gray R, Wagg A, Malone-Lee JG. Differences in detrusor contractile function in women with neuropathic and idiopathic detrusor instability. *Br J Urol* 1997;80:222–6.

5. Fone PD, Vapner JM, Litwiller SE *et al*. Urodynamic findings in the tethered spinal cord syndrome: does surgical release improve bladder function? *J Urol* 1997;157:604–9.

6. Everaert K, Plancke H, Lefevre F, Oosterlinck W. The urodynamic evaluation of neuromodulation in patients with voiding dysfunction. *Br J Urol* 1997;79:702–7.

7. Singh G, Thomas DG. The female tetraplegic: an admission of urological failure. *Br J Urol* 1997;79:708–12.

8. Larsen LD, Chamberlin DA, Khonsari F, Ahlering TE. Retrospective analysis of urologic complications in male patients with spinal cord injury managed with and without indwelling urinary catheters. *Urology* 1997;50(3):418–22.

9. Dasgupta P, Haslam C, Goodwin R, Fowler CJ. The 'Queen Square bladder stimulator': a device for assisting emptying the neurogenic bladder. *Br J Urol* 1997;80:234–7.

10. Cruz F, Guimares M, Silva C, Edite Rio M, Coimbra M, Reis M. Desensitization of bladder sensory fibers by intravesical capsaicin has long lasting clinical and urodynamic effects in patients with hyperactive or hypersensitive bladder dysfunction. *J Urol* 1997;157:585–9.

11. Boucher NR, Thomas DF, Forster D, Smallwood R. A single-centre review of the benefits and complications of sacral anterior root stimulators in patients with spinal cord injury. *Br J Urol* 1997;79 (Suppl 4):47.

12. Schurch B, Rodic B, Jeanmonod D. Posterior sacral rhizotomy and intradural anterior sacral root stimulation for treatment of the spastic bladder in spinal cord injured patients. *J Urol* 1997;157: 610–14.

13. Van Kerrebroeck PhEV, van der Aa HE, Bosch JLHR, Koldewijn EL, Vorsteveld JHC, Debruyne FMJ and the Dutch Study Group on Sacral Anterior Root Stimulation. Sacral rhizotomies and electrical bladder stimulation in spinal cord injury. Part I: Clinical and Urodynamic Analysis. *Eur Urol* 1997;31:263–71.

14. Wielink G, Essink-Bot ML, Van Kerrebroeck PhEV, Rutten FFH and the Dutch Study Group on Sacral Anterior Root Stimulation. Sacral rhizotomies and electrical bladder stimulation in spinal cord injury. Part II: Cost-Effectiveness and Quality of Life Analysis. *Eur Urol* 1997;31:441–6.

15. Probst M, Piechota HJ, Hohenfellner M, Gleason CA, Tanagho EA. Neurostimulation for bladder evacuation: is sacral root stimulation a substitute for microstimulation? *Br J Urol* 1997;79:554–66.

16. ter Meulen PhH, Heesakkers JPFA, Janknegt RA. A study on the feasibility of vesicomyotomy in patients with motor urge incontinence. *Eur Urol* 1997; 32:166–9.

17. Sylora JA, Gonzalez R, Vaughin M, Reinberg Y. Intermittent self-catheterization by quadriplegic patients via a catheterizable Mitrofanoff channel. *J Urol* 1997;157:48–50.

Reconstructive urology

SN Venn and AR Mundy

Institute of Urology and Guy's Hospital, London, UK

Bladder reconstruction

Bladder reconstruction is now an established procedure. The reports published in the last 12 months have mainly concentrated on the morbidity of such procedures, and attempts to quantify morbidity according to the nature of the bowel segment incorporated. Bladder substitution in women, however, continues to feature. It is interesting that it is easier to achieve continence in female patients than in males,[1] but that a much higher proportion of female patients become dependent on catheterization to empty their bladder – a retention state often unnecessarily referred to as 'hypercontinence'.

Metabolic acidosis. There is now no real doubt that enterocystoplasty can cause metabolic acidosis, but whether or not this leads to secondary complications is unclear. Salomon and his group have found no evidence of metabolic dysfunction up to 22 years after a Camey type ileocystoplasty,[2] and Poulsen and colleagues found no evidence of bone mineral loss in elderly men after a Koch ileal bladder substitution procedure, despite the presence of metabolic acidosis.[3] In a similar vein, Kristjansson and co-workers found that, even in the presence of reduced renal function, patients with bladder substitution were able to compensate for metabolic acidosis.[4] Nevertheless, there is evidence from both the UK, USA and, more recently, elsewhere, that metabolic acidosis can lead to loss of growth potential and an increased number of orthopaedic complications in growing children. Thus, in children at least, metabolic acidosis must be carefully sought, closely monitored and adequately treated.

Bowel problems after enterocystoplasty continue to generate interest. Singh and Thomas, as well as others, have found diarrhoea to be a particular problem after enterocystoplasty, especially in patients with neuropathic bladder dysfunction (who have bowel problems anyway), but also in

Highlights in **Reconstructive urology** 1997

WHAT'S IN ?

- Barbagli procedure using buccal mucosa
- Female bladder replacement
- Mainz II recto-sigma pouch

WHAT'S OUT ?

- Bladder mucosa grafting

patients with non-neuropathic problems, such as detrusor instability, in whom bowel problems continue to be a regular source of dissatisfaction after otherwise successful surgery.[5] It must be remembered, however, that one-third of patients with detrusor instability also have smooth muscle dysfunction of the bowel, which causes problems similar to those seen in irritable bowel syndrome. More severe diarrhoea can result from the malabsorption of bile acids and fat; this can occur with or without caeco-ileal reflux, but it is worse when such reflux is present. While the diagnosis is relatively easy to make, treatment is, however, difficult.

Malignancy. Barrington's work in Stephenson's group in Cardiff continues to clarify the nature of malignancy arising after enterocystoplasty.[6] The group has shown that tumours arise in the bladder, rather than the bowel, from adenomatous metaplasia which leads to adenocarcinoma. Tumour development is associated with elevated levels of urinary nitrosamines, which lead to nitrosamine alkylation products that are insufficiently cleared by appropriate scavengers, and are therefore promutagenic. This coupled with an excess of angiogenic growth factors in the urine that act at the suture line between urothelium and bowel leads, eventually, to malignant change. Although the incidence of malignancy after enterocystoplasty is still unknown, all patients are at risk and careful long-term follow-up is essential.

Alternative bladder substitutes. In an attempt to find an alternative to enterocystoplasty, but without resorting to synthetic bladder substitutes, Probst *et al.* investigated the use of an acellular matrix graft.[7] This was a fascinating study, mainly in experimental pathology, which reflects the continuing search for alternative materials for bladder substitution. It is a direction that is more likely to lead to a satisfactory result than the 'plastic bladder'.

Ureterosigmoidostomy is back in favour.[8] At national and international meetings, several groups have reported extremely favourably on their experience of the Mainz modification of the ureterosigmoidostomy (Figure 1) in patients in whom other continent diversion or orthotopic reconstruction is unrealistic. The procedure has the advantage that it avoids the need for catheterization and, furthermore, it is not dependent on the creation of the continence mechanism that is a constant source of problems with most other continent diversion procedures. The largest group of patients for whom this procedure would appear to be most suitable are those requiring a cysto-urethrectomy for transitional cell carcinoma of the bladder. The procedure is obviously equally suitable for men and women.

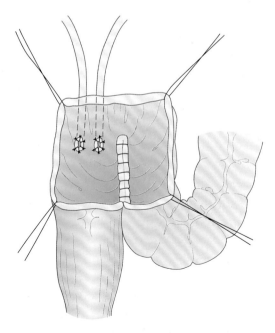

Figure 1 The Mainz II recto-sigma pouch – a modification of the ureterosigmoidostomy.

Urethroplasty

At the recent Reconstructive Urology Symposium held in London, UK, there was almost universal agreement that buccal mucosa is the 'in' material for substitution urethroplasty. Nonetheless, if the bed for a graft is uncertain, a flap would clearly be a better option and, obviously, if an anastomotic urethroplasty is possible then it remains the treatment of choice. However, as substitution urethroplasty is more commonly indicated, there is a large role for buccal mucosa. Almost everyone who has used buccal mucosa has found it easy to harvest, easy to work with and with a reliability of take that gives it an edge over any other form of free graft, especially bladder mucosa. Whether or not the long-term results will be as good remains to be seen, but so far, with 3 years' experience, it appears to be at least as good as the alternatives and better than most. It is particularly to be recommended for strictures due to balanitis xerotica et obliterans, as genital skin urethroplasty in patients with this disease is almost invariably followed by recurrence of the disease in the graft itself.[9]

The other development in substitution urethroplasty is the Barbagli procedure (Figure 2). This involves placing the stricturotomy at 12 o'clock, in the dorsal midline, rather than at 6 o'clock, in the ventral midline. A dorsal midline stricturotomy bleeds far less than a ventral midline stricturotomy, which makes the operation easier from that point of view. It also allows the graft to be fixed firmly onto the corpora cavernosa and the urethra to be fixed firmly to the graft, which is a considerable advantage over graft fixation at 6 o'clock. On the other hand, further back in the bulbar urethra, which is probably the most common site for bulbar urethroplasty, where the dorsal vein complex rather than the corpora cavernosa separates the urethra from the pubic symphysis, the bed is not as good and the procedure is more difficult. Nonetheless, this technique is a useful addition to our armamentarium.

Artificial urinary sphincter

It is perhaps surprising that, after nearly 25 years, there is still only one artificial urinary sphincter on the market – the American Medical Systems model. The AMS800 has now been available in more or less its present form for more than a decade. While expensive, it is an effective device – though it may have mechanical problems in the long term and a tendency towards

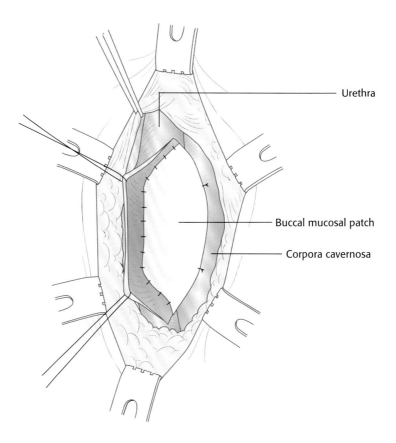

Figure 2 The Barbagli procedure for substitution urethroplasty.

infective complications in the short term. A recent report of a 10-year follow-up of over 60 patients attests to the satisfactory continence rate achieved with this device, but confirms the high revision rate, which effectively fixes the life expectancy of the device at 10 years.[10] Although these results are more pessimistic than the findings of other groups with long-term experience, they are generally in line with experience of others. Most people would conclude that there is probably a better solution to the problem of intractable sphincter weakness incontinence and continuing research into such alternatives is worthwhile.

References

1. Coloby P, France P, Tobisu KI, Kakizoe T. Othotopic ileal neobladder in female patients with bladder cancer. 5-year experience. *J Urol* 1997;157(Suppl 4):383.

2. Salomon L, Lugagne PM, Herve JM, Barre P, Lebret T, Botto H. No evidence of metabolic disorders 10 to 22 years after Camey Type 1 ileo-enterocystoplasty. *J Urol* 1997;157:2104–6.

3. Poulsen AL, Overgaard K, Steven K. Bone metabolism following bladder substitution with the ileal urethral Koch reservoir. *Br J Urol* 1997;79:339–47.

4. Kristjansson A, Davidsson T, Mansson W. Metabolic alterations at different levels of renal function following continent urinary diversion through colonic segments. *J Urol* 1997;157:2099–103.

5. Singh G, Thomas DG. Bowel problems after enterocystoplasty. *Br J Urol* 1997;79:328–32.

6. Barrington JW, Jones A, James D, Smith S, Stephenson TP. Antioxidant deficiency following clam enterocystoplasty. *Br J Urol* 1997;80:238–42.

7. Probst M, Dahiya R, Carrier S, Tanagho EA. Reproduction of functional smooth muscle tissue and partial bladder replacement. *Br J Urol* 1997;79:505–15.

8. Nawrocki J, Venn SN, Mundy AR. The Mainz type ureterosigmoidostomy: a valuable salvage procedure for continent diversion. *Br J Urol* 1997;79(Suppl 4):14.

9. Nawrocki J, Venn SN, Mundy AR. Urethroplasty for balanitis xerotica et obliterans. *Br J Urol* 1997;79(Suppl 4):19.

10. Fulford SCV, Sutton C, Bales G, Hickling M, Stephenson TP. The fate of the 'modern' artificial urinary sphincter with a follow-up of more than 10 years. *Br J Urol* 1997;79:713–16.

Stone disease & minimally invasive surgery

FX Keeley and DA Tolley
Scottish Lithotriptor Centre, Edinburgh, UK

Although few noteworthy advances in the treatment of stone disease have been seen in the past year, previous progress has been consolidated. In contrast, the field of laparoscopic surgery is evolving and a more prominent role in general urological practice is being sought.

Laparoscopic surgery

The boundaries of the laparoscopic approach are being stretched, as evidenced by reports of laparoscopically assisted penile revascularization[1] and laparoscopic nephropexy.[2] In addition, a recent study of extended laparoscopic pelvic lymph node dissection in staging prostate cancer failed to show any advantage over modified lymph node dissection.[3] As the results confirmed, because pre-operative PSA, clinical stage and Gleason sum can reliably predict the likelihood of lymph node metastases, this procedure has a limited role. Taken together, these reports do not encourage the use of laparoscopic techniques in general urological practice.

In contrast, several centres have reported their initial experience with hand-assisted laparoscopic surgery, which may ultimately have a significant impact on general urological practice.[4,5] Specially designed sleeves have been devised, which allow the surgeon to insert and withdraw his hand in the abdomen without loss of pneumoperitoneum. These devices widen the horizons for inexperienced, as well as experienced, laparoscopic surgeons. Indeed, surgeons learning laparoscopic techniques may be encouraged to use this device until they are more comfortable with the procedure. In addition, an experienced laparoscopic surgeon may reasonably take on more complex procedures, such as donor nephrectomy, nephro-ureterectomy and, perhaps, radical nephrectomy to remove a tumour. Furthermore, the 7–8 cm incision necessary to insert the sleeve can be used to remove the specimen without the need for morcellation.

Jacobs *et al.*[6] reported a personal series of 70 donor nephrectomies performed laparoscopically. At the end of the procedure, a midline incision

Highlights in **Stone disease & minimally invasive surgery** *1997*

WHAT'S NEW ?

- Hand-assisted laparoscopy
- Laparoscopic radical nephrectomy
- Laparoscopic adrenalectomy
- Guidelines for treatment of ureteric stones
- Models for endourology training
- Orthopaedic applications of SWL

WHAT'S IN ?

- Laparoscopic donor nephrectomy
- Mechanical endoscopic lithotriptors
- Holmium laser
- Percutaneous nephrolithotomy for large lower pole stones
- *In situ* SWL for ureteric stones
- Percutaneous varicocele embolization
- Ureteroscopic treatment of upper tract tumours

WHAT'S OUT ?

- Open stone surgery
- Laparoscopic pelvic lymph node dissection
- Laparoscopic varicocelectomy

was made to retrieve the kidney. Warm ischaemia time was greater in the laparoscopic group than in a historical series of open donor nephrectomy, but operative times and graft survival were comparable. This is a procedure with great potential, as it may increase the number of relatives willing to donate a kidney. There is, however, concern among urologists that general surgeons may be tempted to perform these procedures.

Another technique on the horizon is laparoscopic radical nephrectomy. Ono *et al.* reported a series of 25 patients with tumours ranging in size from 3 to 7 cm and a low complication rate.[7] The obvious drawback of this procedure, however, was the average operative time of 5.3 hours.

Adrenalectomy is another procedure that may lend itself to the laparoscopic approach. Terachi *et al.* reported their initial 100 cases this year and state that the operative times, excluding the first 10 cases, are comparable with those for open surgery, but with a shorter convalescence period.[8] In contrast, laparoscopic varicocelectomy has been supplanted by percutaneous embolization as the minimally invasive procedure of choice for the treatment of varicoceles.[9]

Training in endourology

Changes in urological training brought about by the Calman ruling in the UK, have drastically shortened training schemes; moreover, restrictions on the number of hours that trainees spend in hospital further limit the time each trainee spends operating. This time pressure has placed a premium on efficiency within training programmes. In order to address this need, several models have become available on which trainees can perform ureteroscopy, percutaneous surgery or prostate resection. These models can be used to learn and practise basic endoscopic skills, as well as to assess competence.

Several presentations on the subject of training were made at the 15th World Congress of Endourology in Edinburgh, UK,[10] all of which had the same underlying point: it is inappropriate, in the late 1990s, for a trainee to learn basic surgical skills for the first time in the operating theatre. Time pressures on theatre lists, the rising threat of litigation and closer scrutiny by managers will ensure that this does not happen in future. Training someone to perform their first ureteroscopic procedure, for example, requires a considerable amount of time (a commodity which is unfortunately in short supply in most theatres) and even more patience. If, however, the trainee has already performed a few dozen procedures on a model, several of which were supervised by the trainer, everyone else in the room may be unaware that this is his first 'real' case. The old surgical maxim 'see one, do one, teach one' is likely to be superseded by 'see one, simulate a few dozen, do one'.

Ureteric stones

The American Urological Association guidelines panel recently reported their findings on the treatment of ureteral stones, following a review of 526 reports published world-wide from 1966 to 1996.[11] Their recommendations, which should not surprise urologists in the UK, are that:

- observation should be the first option for stones 5 mm or smaller in the lower ureter
- *in situ* shock wave lithotripsy (SWL) should be the first-line treatment for stones 1 cm or smaller in the upper ureter, using ureteroscopy and percutaneous removal as salvage procedures
- stones in the lower ureter should be treated by ureteroscopy or SWL, depending on availability and patient preference
- open ureterolithotomy should be used only as a salvage procedure or in unusual circumstances.

The issue of SWL versus ureteroscopy in the treatment of upper ureteric stones was the subject of a formal debate at the recent Societe Internationale de Urologie meeting in Montreal, Canada. In conclusion, Dr Michael Marberger confirmed that a trial of SWL should be offered to a patient first, provided that all the options are available. While it was generally agreed that some centres can achieve very high success rates for proximal ureteric stones using flexible ureteroscopes and the holmium laser, the average urologist usually does not have the necessary expertise and/or equipment. This may, perhaps, change in the future with improvements in training and greater access to technology.

Ureteroscopic instruments

Pursuit of the ideal endoscopic lithotriptor over the past 20 years has covered a wide range of technologies from electrohydraulic (EHL), ultrasonic and mechanical to pulsed-dye and holmium:YAG laser. To date, the holmium laser appears to be the most effective and versatile method, resulting in an 89% stone-free rate following ureteroscopic treatment of intrarenal calculi.[12,13] In addition, in a retrospective comparison of holmium versus EHL for ureteric stones, Teichman *et al.* reported a higher stone-free rate (94% versus 56%) following holmium laser lithotripsy when compared with EHL.[14] They also noted better visibility and less propulsion of fragments with the holmium laser.

Elashry *et al.* proved statistically what most people in the field of endourology have suspected: in the case of ureteroscopes, smaller is better.[15] They compared a 7.5 F flexible ureteroscope (Karl Storz) with a 9.3 F flexible ureteroscope (Olympus) in terms of the need for ureteric dilatation, postoperative pain and successful treatment outcome. The smaller ureteroscope required significantly less ureteric dilatation and caused less postoperative pain; however, they found no difference in success rates.

Endoscopic treatment of upper tract tumours

The efficacy of endoscopic treatment of upper tract transitional cell carcinoma was reported in a series of 41 upper tracts in 38 patients, in which 68% were rendered tumour-free.[16] The recurrence rate was 29%. None of the recurrences was of a higher grade and no local or metastatic progression was found. Adverse prognostic factors to predict incomplete treatment and recurrence included multifocality, high grade and a tumour over 1.5 cm in size. In patients with low-grade, small tumours, the likelihood of having no evidence of disease at the most recent follow-up was greater than 90%. The authors stressed that accurate grading and staging is essential, and that patients undergoing endoscopic treatment need regular endoscopic follow-up, in the same way as patients with transitional cell carcinoma of the bladder. Adjuvant mitomycin C following endoscopic treatment is well tolerated, but its efficacy remains undetermined.[17]

Treatment of renal stones

The Lower Pole Study Group have been conducting a randomized, prospective study of SWL versus percutaneous nephrolithotomy (PCNL) for lower pole stones.[18] An interim analysis, reported by Dr Jim Lingeman, showed that PCNL has a higher stone-free rate (94% versus 42%) and a lower re-treatment rate than SWL. However, PCNL has a higher complication rate than SWL (27% versus 16%) and a longer length of hospital stay (2.95 days versus 0.04 days) is required. This study should make a significant contribution to our management of lower pole stones. In addition, the cost analysis for the two groups is of great interest: SWL is cheaper per treatment, but much more expensive per stone-free patient.[19] Nevertheless, Dr Lingeman's enthusiasm for PCNL is unlikely to be adopted in the UK, because of constraints on theatre time and the fact that SWL costs so much less in the UK than it does in the USA.

Shock wave lithotripsy

Haupt recently reviewed the orthopaedic applications of SWL, which include loosening prosthetic joints before replacement, and the treatment of tendonitis and non-union after fractures.[20] SWL has a potential role in the treatment of patients for whom conservative measures, such as physiotherapy and steroid injections, have failed, as it may avoid the need for surgery. Success rates in limited clinical series have been approximately 60–90%.

References

1. Trombetta C, Liguori G, Siracusano S, Savoca G, Belgrano E. Laparoscopically assisted penile revascularization for vasculogenic impotence: 2 additional cases. *J Urol* 1997;158:1783–6.

2. Fornara P, Doehn C, Jocham D. Laparoscopic nephropexy: 3-year experience. *J Urol* 1997;158:1679–83.

3. Stone NN, Stock RG, Unger P. Laparoscopic pelvic lymph node dissection for prostate cancer: comparison of the extended and modified techniques. *J Urol* 1997;158:1891–4.

4. Keeley FX Jr, Sharma NK, Tolley DA. Hand-assisted laparoscopic nephroureterectomy. *J Urol* 1997;157(Suppl):1565A.

5. Wolf JS Jr, Nakada SY, Moon TD. Hand-assisted laparoscopic nephrectomy: comparison to standard laparoscopic nephrectomy. *J Endourol* 1997;11(Suppl):S129 (Abstract).

6. Jacobs SC, Cho E, Bartlett ST, Flowers JL. A one-year experience with laparoscopic living donor nephrectomy. *J Endourol* 1997;11(Suppl):S128 (Abstract).

7. Ono Y, Katoh N, Kinukawa T, Watsuura O, Ohshima S. Laparoscopic radical nephrectomy: The Nagoya experience. *J Urol* 1997;158:719–23.

8. Terachi T, Matsuda T, Terai A *et al.* Transperitoneal laparoscopic adrenalectomy: experience in 100 patients. *J Endourol* 1997;11:361–5.

9. Feneley MR, Pal MK, Nockler IB, Hendry WF. Retrograde embolization and causes of failure in the primary treatment of varicocele. *Br J Urol* 1997;80:642–6.

10. Moussa SA, Pye SD, Gordon E. A model for percutaneous access. *J Endourol* 1997;11(Suppl):S139 (Abstract).

11. Segura JW, Preminger GM, Assimos DG *et al*. Ureteral stones clinical guidelines panel summary report on the management of ureteral calculi. *J Urol* 1997;158:1915–21.

12. Fabrizio MD, Behari A, Bagley DH. Ureteroscopic management of intrarenal calculi. *J Urol* 1998;In press.

13. Grasso M, Conlin M, Bagley DH. Ureteroscopic treatment of large (> 2 cm) upper urinary tract calculi: multicenter experience. *J Endourol* 1997;11(Suppl): S97(Abstract).

14. Teichman JMH, Rao RD, Rogenes VJ, Harris M. Ureteroscopic management of ureteral calculi: electrohydraulic versus holmium:YAG lithotripsy. *J Urol* 1997;158:1357–61.

15. Elashry OM, Elbahnasy AM, Rao GS, Nakada SY, Clayman RV. Flexible ureteroscopy: Washington University experience with the 9.3F and 7.5F flexible ureteroscopes. *J Urol* 1997;157: 2074–80.

16. Keeley FX Jr, Bibbo M, Bagley DH. Ureteroscopic treatment and surveillance of upper urinary tract transitional cell carcinoma. *J Urol* 1997;157:1560–5.

17. Keeley FX Jr, Bagley DH. Adjuvant mitomycin C following endoscopic treatment of upper tract transitional cell carcinoma. *J Urol* 1997;158:2074–7.

18. Lingeman JE for the Lower Pole Study Group. Prospective randomized trial of extracorporeal shock wave lithotripsy and percutaneous nephrostolithotomy for lower pole nephrolithiasis; initial long-term follow up. *J Endourol* 1997;11(Suppl):S95 (Abstract).

19. Nakada SY, Saywell RM, Lingeman JE, Woods JR, Robinson RL. Cost analysis of percutaneous nephrostolithotomy and extracorporeal shock wave lithotripsy for the treatment of lower pole nephrolithiasis. *J Endourol* 1997;11(Suppl):S146(Abstract).

20. Haupt G. Use of extracorporeal shock waves in the treatment of pseudoarthosis, tendinopathy and other orthopedic diseases. *J Urol* 1997;158: 4–11.

Urinary tract infection

GR Sant

Department of Urology, Tufts University School of Medicine, Boston, USA

Over the past year, particular interest has focused on non-bacterial infections and inflammatory diseases of the urinary tract, such as interstitial cystitis and non-bacterial prostatitis. Studies have also continued into the pathogenesis, treatment and prevention of recurrent bacterial cystitis.

Bacterial cystitis

The diagnosis of bacterial cystitis has become more 'user-friendly', with dip-stick culture tests providing a rapid method of isolating pathogens. Nevertheless, empirical therapy is more cost effective than culture in uncomplicated urinary tract infection (UTI) in women. The organisms causing UTIs have not changed over the past 2 decades and *Escherichia coli* is still the most commonly implicated organism. Antibiotic susceptibility patterns have, however, altered dramatically with the emergence of resistance to ampicillin.[1] In addition, the fluoroquinolones, which had been extremely effective against Gram-negative enteric pathogens, are no longer universally active and pathogens, such as *Pseudomonas* and *Enterococcus*, may be resistant.

Faecal–perineal–urethral hypothesis. This hypothesis to explain the cause of UTI with enteric bacteria is supported by longitudinal studies of serotyping and urovirulence factors. Pulsed-gel electrophoresis, a precise genetic technique, has been used to identify isolates of *E. coli* in the urine and faeces of patients with cystitis. This has confirmed the hypothesis that strains of *E. coli* in the rectal flora are a reservoir for infection of the lower urinary tract.[2]

Antibiotic prophylaxis. Long-term, low-dose oral antibiotic prophylaxis is the mainstay of treatment for women with recurrent bacterial cystitis. However, ciprofloxacin prophylaxis following sexual intercourse has proved to be as effective as daily prophylaxis, and has the major advantage of requiring only one-third of the quantity of drug.[3]

The increase in the number of transrectal prostate biopsies performed as a result of PSA testing led to a retrospective review of 4439 biopsies to determine the rate of symptomatic UTI following the procedure.[4] Patients were routinely treated with ciprofloxacin, 500 mg twice daily, for 8 doses beginning the day before biopsy. Only five cases of symptomatic UTI occurred. Thus, routine oral fluoroquinolone antibiotic prophylaxis is recommended for patients undergoing transrectal prostate biopsies.

Vaccine. In a double-blind, placebo-controlled, Phase II study, a multi-strain vaccine was administered as a vaginal suppository to 91 women with recurrent bacterial cystitis.[5] Patients received three vaginal suppositories at weekly intervals without serious adverse effects. Vaginal mucosal immunization enhances resistance to UTIs in susceptible patients and is, therefore, a promising approach to the prevention of recurrent cystitis in women.

Nitric oxide synthase activity. The role of nitric oxide in many human diseases is being elucidated. Inducible nitric oxide synthase is the major nitric oxide synthase isoform found in urinary neutrophils. A significant (43-fold) increase in nitric oxide synthase activity has been found to occur in UTI,[6] which does not fall until 6–10 days after the start of antibiotic treatment. This may well explain the delay in irritative voiding symptom relief that frequently follows bacteriological cure of UTI.

Fosfomycin tromethamine is a phosphonic acid bactericidal agent with *in-vitro* activity against most urinary tract pathogens. A new formulation of fosfomycin, as the oral tromethamine salt, has a bioavailability of 34–41%, a mean elimination half-life of 5.7 hours, and is primarily excreted unchanged in the urine. Following a single 3 g oral dose, peak urine concentrations occur within 4 hours. Side-effects are mainly gastrointestinal. The efficacy of fosfomycin, its single-dose administration and a favourable pregnancy category rating make it a useful antibiotic in the treatment of acute uncomplicated UTIs.[7]

Highlights in **Urinary tract infection** *1997*

WHAT'S IN ?

- New classification of prostatitis
- Pharmacological treatment of interstitial cystitis
  - sodium pentosan polysulphate
  - intravesical BCG and hyaluronic acid
  - hydroxyzine
  - L-arginine
- Molecular biological techniques for identifying urinary pathogens
- Nitric oxide and nitric oxide synthase in bladder inflammation
- The O'Leary-Sant symptom index for interstitial cystitis

WHAT'S OUT ?

- Major surgery for interstitial cystitis
- Long-term antibiotic treatment of uncomplicated cystitis
- Meares-Stamey classification of prostatitis

Interstitial cystitis

Interstitial cystitis is an enigmatic bladder disorder of unknown origin. Modern molecular biological techniques, such as the polymerase chain reaction (PCR), have been used to look for a possible bacterial cause, using nested PCR assays for conserved bacterial 16S rRNA genes. However, multiple reports suggest that a primary bacterial aetiology for interstitial cystitis is unlikely. A recent review concluded that laboratory culture, light and electron microscopy, and molecular strategies to detect micro-organisms and viruses in interstitial cystitis have failed to identify an infectious aetiology.[8]

Nitric oxide synthase activity. Data on nitric oxide and urinary nitric oxide synthase activity in interstitial cystitis are conflicting; a previous study from

Scandinavia reported increased activity,[9] while a more recent study showed decreased activity.[10] In this small, self-controlled, non-placebo study, the oral nitric oxide donor, L-arginine (a substrate for nitric oxide synthase), 1.5 g/day for 6 months, was given to 10 patients with interstitial cystitis. The results showed a decrease in abdominal and vaginal pain scores, providing evidence that oral L-arginine improves symptoms related to interstitial cystitis.

Hydroxyzine is now an accepted drug for the symptomatic treatment of interstitial cystitis, especially in patients with documented allergies and/or evidence of bladder mast cell activation on bladder biopsy.[11]

Abnormality of the bladder epithelium. Bladder epithelial abnormality (either primary or secondary) has been postulated as a cause of interstitial cystitis. However, changes in the levels of urinary glycosaminoglycans, either total or individual, have not been found in interstitial cystitis.[12] Although anti-epithelial cell autoantibodies are present in the urine of patients with interstitial cystitis, they are unlikely to be a primary cause of the disease.[13] Following ingestion of fluorescein, urinary excretion is significantly ($p < 0.05$) lower in patients with interstitial cystitis compared with controls, and this may be a useful marker of altered membrane permeability.[14]

Drugs that target this putative membrane abnormality are being increasingly used to treat interstitial cystitis. Sulphated polysaccharides (e.g. sodium pentosan polysulphate), administered orally and intravesically, are effective long-term treatment for interstitial cystitis. A meta-analysis of the published data concluded that oral pentosan polysulphate is more effective than placebo in the treatment of pain, urgency and frequency, but not the nocturia, associated with interstitial cystitis.[15]

Symptom index. The O'Leary-Sant Index is a validated symptom index that has been developed to measure lower urinary tract symptoms and their significance in patients with interstitial cystitis.[16] This index holds promise for disease monitoring (similar to the International Prostate Symptom Score) and assessment of new therapies in clinical trials in which reliable, validated and reproducible treatment outcomes are essential.

Other treatments. Intravesical hyaluronic acid has been shown to be effective in patients with interstitial cystitis refractory to standard treatment.[17] The response was not durable and placebo-controlled studies are underway to determine the true efficacy of hyaluronic acid, as well as to establish optimum dosing and maintenance regimens. In a blinded, placebo-controlled study, intravesical BCG was shown to be a well-tolerated and effective treatment with durable responses.[18] A small study demonstrated that intravesical pentosan polysulphate is an effective and well-tolerated option for the treatment of interstitial cystitis.[19]

Systemic disease. Many patients with interstitial cystitis complain of symptoms suggestive of systemic diseases (e.g. autoimmune diseases). Current data suggest that there is significant symptom overlap between fibromyalgia and interstitial cystitis; patients with interstitial cystitis have a diffuse increase in peripheral nociception similar to that seen in fibromyalgia.[20]

Drug-induced interstitial cystitis. The non-steroidal anti-inflammatory drug, tiaprofenic acid, is now known to cause cystitis.[21] Most cases are reversible on withdrawal of the drug, although 10% of patients experience residual symptoms. On cystoscopy and biopsy, the findings are similar to interstitial cystitis and, as a result, many patients undergo extensive urological surgery for presumed chronic interstitial cystitis. This highlights the importance of taking a full drug history in patients with symptoms of cystitis.

Pain. Urological, gastrointestinal or gynaecological pain is a cardinal symptom of interstitial cystitis, which previous studies have shown to be associated with increased bladder innervation and expression of neuropeptides. Immunostaining has demonstrated increased expression of nerve growth factor in the urothelium of patients with interstitial cystitis and, more markedly, in patients with idiopathic sensory urgency.[22] Thus, treatment with anti-nerve growth factor may be a rational and effective treatment for painful bladder conditions.

Chronic prostatitis syndromes

The prostatitis syndromes are characterized by irritative voiding symptoms, pain (perineal, bladder, scrotal and perirectal) and varying degrees of sexual dysfunction. The Meares-Stamey classification uses segmented urine cultures – VB 1, VB 2, EPS and VB 3 – to distinguish chronic bacterial prostatitis from non-bacterial prostatitis and prostatodynia. A simple and cost-effective screen for prostatitis, involving the culture and microscopy of urine before and after prostatic massage (the pre- and post-massage test; PPMT) led to the same diagnosis as standard testing.[23] The PPMT test is, therefore, a potentially attractive tool for urologists, as well as family physicians, dealing with patients with symptoms suggestive of prostatitis.

Granulomatous prostatitis was identified in 9 of 12 (75%) patients undergoing radical cystoprostatectomy for bladder cancer following therapy with intravesical BCG, and acid-fast bacilli were identified in 7 of these 9 patients.[24] The incidence of granulomatous prostatitis after intravesical BCG therapy is far greater than the reported incidence of symptomatic granulomatous prostatitis.

Classification. A new classification of chronic prostatitis has been promoted by the National Institutes of Health in the USA. Chronic bacterial prostatitis, diagnosed by positive identification of bacteria in the prostatic fluid, is found in only 5–10% of patients with symptoms of prostatitis. Non-bacterial prostatitis and prostatodynia are now classified as chronic pelvic pain of undermined aetiology, with non-bacterial prostatitis having a putative inflammatory cause and prostatodynia being non-inflammatory.[23] This new classification should lead to a better understanding and stratification of patients with prostatitis.

Prevalence. The community prevalence of chronic prostatitis is not insignificant and a report from Rochester, Minnesota, USA, suggests a prevalence of 1.5%.[25] There is emerging evidence that men with interstitial cystitis are often misdiagnosed as suffering from non-bacterial prostatitis or prostatodynia.[23] If this is indeed true, the female preponderance of interstitial cystitis may well be reduced in the future.

Treatment. Chronic non-bacterial prostatitis and prostatodynia are difficult entities to treat, mainly because their aetiologies and pathogenesis are not well understood. A preliminary study of four patients treated with finasteride has, however, showed encouraging results.[26] Other researchers are beginning to investigate the use of treatments for interstitial cystitis (e.g. sodium pentosan polysulphate, tricyclic antidepressants) in these patients.[23] The true role of these treatments for non-bacterial prostatitis and prostatodynia can, however, only be established by prospective, randomized, placebo-controlled studies.

References

1. Bacheller CD, Bernstein JM. Urinary tract infections. *Med Clin North Am* 1997;81:71.

2. Yamamoto S, Tsukamoto T, Terai A, Kurazono H, Takeda Y, Yoshida O. Genetic evidence supporting the fecal-perineal-urethral hypothesis in cystitis caused by *Escherichia coli*. *J Urol* 1997;157:1127–9.

3. Melekos MD, Asbach HW, Gerharz E, Zarakovitis IE, Weingaertner K, Naber KG. Post-intercourse versus daily ciprofloxacin prophylaxis for recurrent urinary tract infections in premenopausal women. *J Urol* 1997;157:935–9.

4. Sieber PR, Rommel FM, Agusta VE, Breslin JA, Huffnagle HW, Harpster LE. Antibiotic prophylaxis in ultrasound guided prostate biopsy. *J Urol* 1997;157:2199–200.

5. Uheling DT, Hopkins WJ, Balish E, Xing Y, Heisey DM. Vaginal mucosal immunization for recurrent urinary tract infection: phase II clinical trial. *J Urol* 1997;157:2049–52.

6. Wheeler MA, Smith SD, Garcia-Cardena G, Nathan CF, Weiss RM, Sessa WC. Bacterial infection induces nitric oxide synthase in human neutrophils. *J Clin Invest* 1997;99:110–16.

7. Patel SS, Balfour JA, Bryson HM. Fosfomycin tromethamine. A review of its antibacterial activity, pharmacokinetic properties and therapeutic efficacy as a single-dose oral treatment for acute uncomplicated lower urinary tract infections. *Drugs* 1997;53:637–56.

8. Duncan JL, Schaeffer AJ. Do infectious agents cause interstitial cystitis? Urology 1997;49(Suppl 5A): 48–51.

9. Lundberg JO, Ehren I, Jansson O *et al*. Elevated nitric oxide in the urinary bladder in infectious and noninfectious cystitis. *Urology* 1996;48:700–2.

10. Smith SD, Wheeler MA, Foster HE Jr, Weiss RM. Improvement in interstitial cystitis symptom scores during treatment with oral L-arginine. *J Urol* 1997;158: 703–8.

11. Theoharides TC, Sant GR. Hydroxyzine therapy for interstitial cystitis. *Urology* 1997;49(Suppl 5A): 108–10.

12. Erickson DR, Ordille S, Martin A, Bhavanandan VP. Urinary chondroitin sulfates, heparan sulfate and total sulfated glysosaminoglycans in interstitial cystitis. *J Urol* 1997;157:61–4.

13. Keay S, Zhang CO, Trifillis AL, Hebel JR, Jacobs SC, Warren JW. Urine autoantibodies in interstitial cystitis. *J Urol* 1997;157:1083–7.

14. Buffington CA, Woodworth BE. Excretion of fluorescein in the urine of women with interstitial cystitis. *J Urol* 1997;158:786–9.

15. Hwang P, Auclair B, Beechinor D, Diment M, Einarson TR. Efficacy of pentosan polysulfate in the treatment of interstitial cystitis: a meta-analysis. *Urology* 1997;50:39–43.

16. O'Leary MP, Sant GR, Fowler FJ Jr., Whitmore KE, Spolarich-Kroll J. The interstitial cystitis symptom index and problem index. *Urology* 1997;49(Suppl 5A):58–63.

17. Morales A, Emerson L, Nickel JC. Intravesical hyaluronic acid in the treatment of refractory interstitial cystitis. *Urology* 1997;49(Suppl 5A): 111–13.

18. Peters K, Diokno A, Steinhert B *et al.* The efficacy of intravesical Tice strain Bacillus Calmette-Guerin in the treatment of interstitial cystitis: a double-blind, prospective, placebo-controlled trial. *J Urol* 1997;157:2090–4.

19. Bade JJ, Laseur M, Nieuwenburg A, van der Weele LT, Mensink HJ. A placebo-controlled study of intravesical pentosan polysulfate for the treatment of interstitial cystitis. *Br J Urol* 1997;79: 168–71.

20. Clauw DJ, Schmidt M, Radulovic D, Singer A, Katz P, Bresette J. The relationship between fibromyalgia and interstitial cystitis. *J Psychiatric Res* 1997;31:125–1.

21. Henley MJ, Hariss D, Bishop MC. Cystitis associated with tiaprofenic acid: a survey of British and Irish urologists. *Br J Urol* 1997;79:585–7.

22. Lowe EM, Anand P, Terenghi G, Williams-Chestnut RE, Sinicropi DV, Osborne JL. Increased nerve growth factor levels in the urinary bladder of women with idiopathic sensory urgency and interstitial cystitis. *Br J Urol* 1997;79:572–7.

23. Nickel JC. The Pre and Post Massage Test (PPMT): a simple screen for prostatitis. *Techniques in Urology* 1997;3:38–43.

24. LaFontaine PD, Middleman BR, Graham SD Jr., Sanders WH. Incidence of granulomatous prostatitis and acid-fast bacilli after intravesical BCG therapy. *Urology* 1997;49:363–6.

25. Roberts RO, Jacobsen SJ, Rhodes T, Girman CJ, Guess HA, Lieber MM. A community-based study on the prevalence of prostatitis. *J Urol* 1997;157(Suppl 4):242A.

26. Holm M, Meyhoff HH. Chronic prostatic pain. A new treatment option with finasteride? *Scand J Urol and Nephrol* 1997;31:213–15.

Index

How to order

This *Fast Facts* book is one of a rapidly growing series of concise clinical handbooks.

Current *Fast Facts* titles:
- Benign Gynaecological Disease
- Benign Prostatic Hyperplasia
- Diabetes Mellitus
- Infections Highlights 1997
- Male Erectile Dysfunction
- Prostate Cancer
- Prostate Specific Antigen
- Urology Highlights 1996
- Osteoporosis
- Rheumatology Highlights 1997

For an up-to-date list of other titles in this series or an order form, simply phone or fax:

Phone: +44 (0)1235 523 233
Fax: +44 (0)1235 523 238